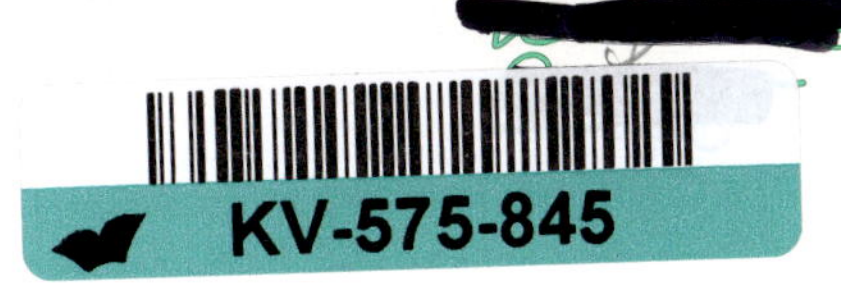

Occupational Therapy in Mental Health

Occupational Therapy in Mental Health:

Principles in Practice

Edited by

Derek W. Scott and Noomi Katz

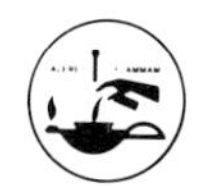

Taylor & Francis

London, New York and Philadelphia

UK Taylor & Francis Ltd. 4 John St, London WC1N 2ET

USA Taylor & Francis Inc., 242 Cherry St, Philadelphia, PA 19106-1906

Library of Congress Cataloging-in-Publication Data

Occupational therapy in mental health: principles in practice, edited by Derek W. Scott and Noomi Katz.
p. cm.
Includes bibliographies and index.
1. Occupational therapy. 2. Mentally ill—Rehabilitation.
I. Scott, Derek W. II. Katz, Noomi.
[DNLM: 1. Mental Disorders—rehabilitation. 2. Occupational Therapy. WM 450.5.020149]
RC487.0253 1988 615.8'5152—dc 19 88-2242
ISBN 0-85066-464-0
ISBN 0-85066-451-9 (pbk.)

Typeset in 11/13 Bembo by
Alresford Typesetting & Design, New Farm Road, Alresford, Hants.

Printed in Great Britain by
Redwood Burn Limited, Trowbridge, Wiltshire.

Contents

Preface

The rationale behind this book was that all occupational therapists with whom I had spoken (from both sides of the Atlantic) felt that a gap existed in the present texts. There seemed a very definite bias towards theoretical discussion rather than the practical application. Additionally, those few books with the emphasis on the mental side generally did not fully address specific problems encountered by occupational therapists. This text hopes to redress the balance.

The potential audience is seen as both students and practising occupational therapists, particularly those who are moving into new areas and need an overview from someone with prior experience. The intention has been for the practical problems as opposed to theoretical frameworks to be emphasized. As contributors come from as far afield as the United Kingdom, the United States, Canada, Australia and Israel, we hope that this will be of use to people world-wide and not merely appeal to a national audience. We have aimed at producing a book which can realistically be purchased by individuals, rather than being a tome destined to a life on the library shelf. When I advertized for contributions I received over thirty suggestions for inclusion. Particularly due to limitations in length, I have had to be selective in choosing topics for inclusion. There had to be disappointments and I deeply thank all potential contributors who had to be left out. Of course there will be claims that a chapter on such-and-such should have been included. It is difficult to satisfy everyone. A wide range of subject matter was chosen including some on established areas and some on developing lines, but by no means are they a representative sample of all OT practice.

It was at this stage that Noomi Katz joined in with the editorial duties. It must also be mentioned that we do not necessarily agree with all views expressed by the contributors. Nor do we expect all readers to agree with the views contained here. One cannot expect the broad spectrum encompassed within occupational therapy to be clear-cut. However, we do hope that any discussions or arguments produced will be productive.

Several people have asked me why I, as a psychologist, decided on this project and had the audacity to edit such a book. Firstly, I have been fortunate in having the benefit and experience of working with many occupational therapists in a variety of psychiatric and mental handicap hospitals. Some of these professionals have been particularly impressive, and to them I owe the inspiration for this venture. Most importantly though, in a time when the human relevance of much psychology is being seriously challenged, I quite simply see the mental health side of occupational therapy as the epitome of applied psychology.

Finally, as the vast majority of occupational therapists are female, we have taken the logical decision to use the female pronoun throughout. We trust that male colleagues will not be offended by this departure from tradition.

Derek W. Scott
November 1987

Chapter 1

Principles and Theoretical Approaches in Practice

Noomi Katz

This introductory chapter aims to provide a frame through which the reader may reflect on the content of the various occupational therapy (OT) applications presented in this book by authors from all over the world. The book is essentially a collection of OT experiences as presented by the authors. Therefore, the intention is here to highlight the unifying elements, and to provide the reader with additional theoretical references in OT for further development and study of OT clinical practice.

Occupational therapy in mental health compasses a wide range of approaches and methods of practice, as this book exemplifies. This fact may be part of OT's attractiveness but also a drawback, as diversity not always leads to systematic and scientific knowledge development. The field of psychiatric OT, although the oldest one in the profession, began only recently to expand and articulate its knowledge base in the form of clearly defined theories or frames of reference which include evaluation instruments, treatment methods and some research to substantiate their merits.

But why do we need theories? Is it not enough to have a philosophy to guide us in practice, and to feel that we do an important job? Obviously it is not enough any more, if it ever was in the past. Mosey (1981, 1986) provides us with a configuration of OT which describes the link between philosophy, theory/research and practice. She suggests a professional model that consists of six elements: (a) philosophical assumptions; (b) an ethical code; (c) a body of knowledge; (d) a domain of concern; (e) the nature and aspects of practice; and (f) legitimate tools.

For the purpose of discussing the OT applications provided in this book, these six elements will be organized into three major sections:

1 philosophical assumptions and ethical codes comprising the principles underlying practice — the art of therapy:

2 a body of knowledge, namely theories, models and frames of reference guiding practice and research — the science of therapy;
3 the domain of concern, aspects of practice and legitimate tools, areas and methods of OT's intervention — the practice of OT.

Reed (1984), in her proposed model, 'adaptation through occupation', presents in a similar manner the relationship between the three elements of philosophy, paradigms and practice (p. 510). These three parts — philosophical principles, scientific theories and service delivery methods — will be briefly presented and each discussed in relation to the various chapters of the book.

Philosophical Principles — The Art of Therapy

The principles of OT in practice are derived from the profession's philosophical foundation and ethics. This philosophical base unites the profession and provides the core beliefs and assumptions of all occupational therapists (OTs) in their clinical work. These principles were first articulated in an article by Meyer in 1922 (republished in 1977) on the philosophy of OT, in which the value of work in adaptation and the balanced use of time were emphasized; they were further developed in numerous additional works into a humanistic, existential but also organismic and pragmatic profession of OT (Yerxa, 1967, 1983; Owen, 1968; Dunning, 1973; Johnson, 1977; King, 1978; Fidler and Fidler, 1978; Fidler, 1981; Bing, 1981, 1986; Allen, 1985; Mosey, 1985).

Among the major principles are the beliefs: (a) in the unity of body and mind; (b) that individuals are entitled to a meaningful existence; (c) that they actualize their sociocultural environment; (d) that individuals have inner needs for occupation with purpose (to be active purposefully in daily living tasks, work and play); and (e) their functional independence in occupation is the major factor in determining their health within their cultural environment.

These beliefs underline the OT principles of collaborating with patients in promoting their independent competent performance, where patients are active participants in the process of therapy, and also have rights to accept or refuse treatment. In the sense of a treatment that involves the patient in task performance, as well as in decision-making at the level of his/her capabilities, one needs a belief in a person as a whole, active and engaged in reality (Engelhardt, 1977, 1986).

Occupational therapy intervention is perceived as providing opportunities in a process of mutual collaboration between patient and therapist, in which patients are involved in purposeful activities of their choice or preference according to their level of competency and environmental demands. This process aims at the individual's renewed adaptation to their cultural environment, or in other words their rehabilitation. In addition, in some areas OT has recently developed an important role in primary prevention by screening for potential risks in adaptation (Mosey, 1986; Parush *et al.*, 1987).

Figure 1.1 provides an illustration of the relationships between these key concepts in OT intervention.

Healthy performances in the areas of occupation are believed to be essential for competent and satisfying adaptation to the environment. Therefore, early screening of infants is important in order to prevent possible difficulties in adaptation. On the other hand, when functional adaptation is disrupted or found to be at risk, rehabilitation is believed to be achieved by renewed participation of the patient in purposeful activity with

Figure 1.1. Relationships of Major OT Concepts in Intervention.

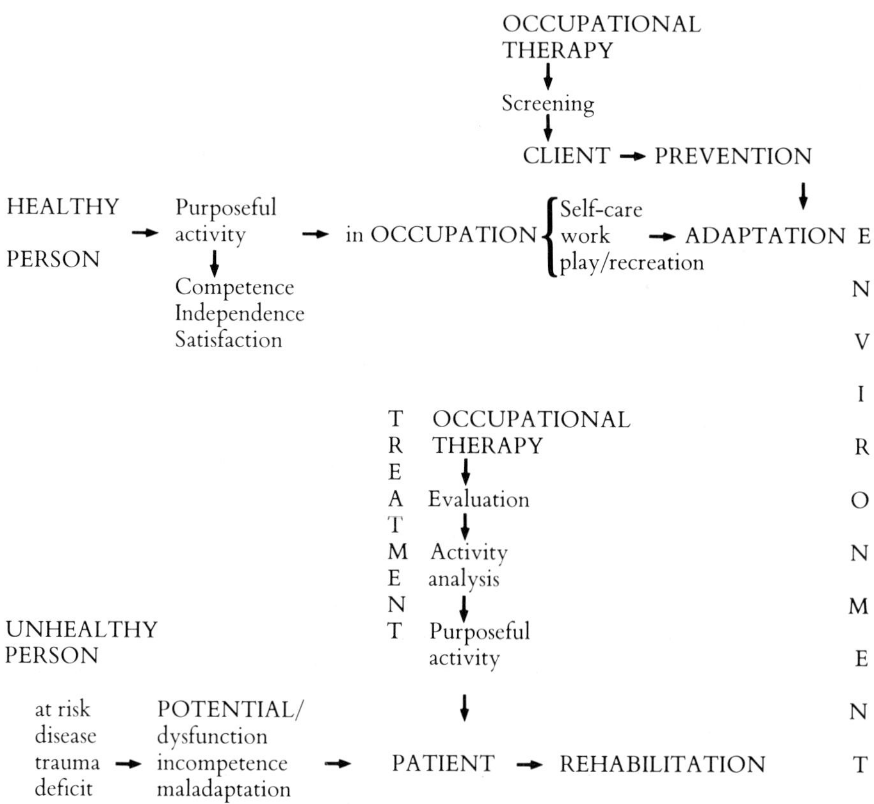

the expert guidance by the occupational therapist in a climate of care. As stated by Yerxa (1980), '. . . a person can be healthy in the sense of being competent in occupational performance . . .' (p. 532). Thus knowledgeable, skilful, creative and humanistic-oriented caring is conceived as the art of therapy; namely, OT's philosophy of practice (Baum, 1980; Gilfoyle, 1980; King, 1980; Yerxa, 1980).

The basic philosophical principles or beliefs are consistently presented in the various chapters of this book. These principles seem to be part of a humanistic and holistic view of man, in which the patient is accepted with respect for his/her rights. If possible the patient is involved in decisions about his treatment goals and methods. Caring and helping relationships are emphasized to enable the patient to achieve self-actualization. The ultimate focus of OT and its unique contribution is the concern for optimal function in occupation with the belief that action and doing are essential for competent performance, independence and satisfaction. Purposeful activity gives meaning to life. Occupational therapy believes in quality of life which can be achieved by every person at the level of his/her capability, given the opportunity, and in enabling experience through adaptation to tasks and environmental demands. The emphasis is on patients' strengths and assets. Occupation and active engagement in this are seen as major factors in humans' normal adaptation, and as the mode of therapy towards rehabilitation of patients in their environment (see Figure 1.1). In addition, throughout the book OT is seen as part of an interdisciplinary health team working together towards patients' rehabilitation with special emphasis on long-term mentally ill patients who have residual deficits.

It appears that the art of therapy which is rooted in OT's philosophy is very clear and powerful, but it provides only the general approach and attitude. Conceptual models based on sound scientific knowledge have to structure the actual clinical practice, in accordance with the spirit of the principles highlighted above. Therefore, in the next section theories, models or frames of reference in OT will be considered.

Theories, Models and Frames of Reference: The Science of Therapy

As the title of this section implies it is concerned with the theoretical base of OT evaluation and intervention, without trying to differentiate between these terms, a debate which is not essential for our purpose. Mosey (1981, 1986) and Reed (1984) conceptualize models and frames of reference differently. Mosey perceives a model as the general configuration in which various frames of reference are included; Reed defines frames of reference as part of philosophy and a variety of models as organizing OT practice. But basically all agree that theoretical approaches for practical professions refer to: (a) sets of concepts; (b) assumptions or postulates; (c) evaluation instruments for assessing a function/dysfunction continuum; and (d) intervention strategies with well defined outcomes which should enable research to demonstrate the effectiveness of the intervention. These theoretical approaches are the scientific links between the philosophy of the profession and its practice.

Historically, however, a profession's development does not always follow a sequence of philosophy-theory-practice, which would imply a *deductive* method, but it may develop *inductively* from practice to theory and checked against its philosophy (Dunning, 1973). More often a profession develops from philosophical assumptions directly into practice, via scientific knowledge from other disciplines to support it at first, and only later develops its own unique scientific theories, a process which is long and dynamic. It seems that for the most part OT followed this path of theory development, which Reynolds (1971) may call the practice-theory-research strategy for scientific knowledge development. Still, there are practices which directly follow a theory outside OT, such as behaviour modification or a humanistic approach, and are applied to OT without any major transformation but in relation to the profession's principles (see Table 1.1).

Occupational therapy in mental health started in the 1920s with Meyer's philosophy derived from moral treatment and applied by Slagle's habit training model of OT (Reed, 1984; Mosey, 1986). This approach was replaced later during the 1930s and through the mid-1950s by more directive relationships between symptoms and activities used in therapy. A major shift in OT in mental health occurred with the influence of psychoanalytic theory which was developed in OT into a psychodynamic approach by Azima and Azima (1959) and Fidler and Fidler (1954, 1963) whose books became OT's major theoretical foundations until the 1970s.

With the changes occurring in society and medicine, OT in mental health developed a variety of additional theoretical approaches such as: (a) Reilly's (1966) occupational behaviour frame of reference; (b) Llorens' (1970a, 1970b) developmental theory called 'facilitating growth and development'; and (c) Mosey's (1970) three frames of reference — analytical, acquisitional and developmental — (called then, object relations, action consequence, and recapitulation of ontogenesis and changed in Mosey's recent (1986) book to a reconciliation of universal issues, role acquisition and recapitulation of ontogenesis, respectively). In addition, Mosey (1973) formulated another acquisitional frame of reference, activities therapy, which was based on learning theories as well as developmental theories and group dynamics, referring mainly to activity groups in OT,

Table 1.1. Theories, Models and Frames of Reference in Mental Health Occupational Therapy According to Chronological Order.

Theories	Major authors
Habit training	Slagle (1920s)
Psychodynamic approach	Azima and Azima (1959)
	Fidler and Fidler (1954, 1963)
Occupational behaviour	Reilly (1966)
Analytical frame of reference	Mosey (1970) 1986*
Acquisitional frame of reference	Mosey (1970) 1986*
Activities therapy	Mosey (1973)
Developmental frame of reference	Mosey (1970) 1986*
Developmental theory	Llorens (1970, 1976)
Sensory integration	King (1974, 1982)
Adaptive or functional	Fidler (1978–1984)
performance**	Mosey (1970, 1986)
Human occupation model	Kielhofner and colleagues (since 1980)
Cognitive disabilities theory	Allen (1982, 1985)
Direct application of psychological theories to OT in mental health	
	Presented by:
Behaviour modification	Briggs *et al.* (1979)
	Sieg (1974)
	Tiffany (1983)
	Wilson (1983)
Humanistic approaches	Briggs *et al.* (1979)
	Tiffany (1983)
	Wilson (1983)

Notes:) Republished with some changes.*
**Not published as such by the two authors — integrated by others (Clark, 1979; Denton, 1987).

while King's (1974) application of sensory integration theory (Ayers, 1972) for schizophrenic patients is an example of a developmental frame of reference which was not developed primarily for mental health, and limits itself to one diagnosis only.

Based on Fidler and Fidler (1963, 1978) and Mosey (1970), Clarke (1979) describes an adaptive performance theoretical framework integrating concepts of doing and becoming with adaptive skills. This approach is further described by Fidler (1981, 1982, 1984) with concepts of lifestyle performance and psychiatric rehabilitation. More recently, Denton (1987) termed it a functional performance frame of reference including all of OT's domain of concern competence components (psychological, social, cognitive, motor and sensory integration; Fidler, 1982; Katz, 1985).

Finally, in the 1980s two major theoretical approaches were published. Firstly, is the model of human occupation (Kielhofner, 1980a, 1980b, 1983, 1985; Kielhofner and Burke, 1980; Kielhofner *et al.*, 1980; Barris *et al.*, 1983) which was derived from the occupational behaviour frame of reference (Reilly, 1966, 1969, 1974), and based on concepts from psychosocial and anthropological theories as well as general system theory. Secondly, is cognitive disability theory developed by Allen (1982, 1985) in a gradual process since the mid-1970s, and is based primarily on cognitive and biological concepts derived from Piaget and the neurosciences, as well as the concept of activity analysis in OT focusing on the understanding of dysfunctional behaviour related to cognitive disabilities in patients' task performance. Table 1.1 lists OT theories in mental health with their major authors according to chronological order.

In evaluating the heuristic value of the different theories mentioned, large differences among them appear. Most publications in the profession's journals of the 1980s, regarding evaluation instruments and intervention methods, are related to the occupational behaviour frame of reference and/or the model of human occupation. Previous approaches such as Fidler's psychodynamic, Lloren's developmental theory, or Mosey's frame of reference did not produce much research, and even in their new form presented again in Mosey's (1986) book, almost no research is cited to support them. Most relevant existing projective instruments and performance scales are assembled in Hemphill (1982), but only some of them with initial research data.

In relation to King's application of sensory integration, few studies were conducted in the late 1970s, but since then development seemed to stop, even though Ross and Burdick (1981) published a sensory integration training manual and assessment tools such as King's (1982) Person Symbol assessment tool, and Schroeder *et al.'s* (1982) Adult Psychiatric Sensory Integration Evaluation (SBC) were described in mental health. Recently, Denton (1987) described it as one of four OT frames of reference for mental health in her workbook.

Finally, cognitive disability seems to take its place with the publication of Allen's book (1985) which includes theory, practice and initial research, and further works and studies by Denton (1987), Katz *et al.* (in press), Levy (1987) and Mayer (1988), as well as Allen's (1987) Eleanor Clarke Slagle Lecture.

All approaches mentioned above are theories or models of OT, namely bodies of knowledge uniquely articulated for guiding OT practice and research. These theories are in various stages of development and acceptance in the profession, but as suggested by Reynolds (1971), it is expected that as empirical support increases confidence in them will also increase. With the growing research activity in OT, it is expected that its theoretical foundation will be substantiated and expanded, leading to more direct guidance for practice. In the meantime however, the practice of OT mental health still shows direct applications of theories from psychology with any OT transformation, and an array of methods derived from other disciplines and applied to OT. Some of these are evident in the book and will be discussed later.

Theories in Mental Health

The intent of this section is to present briefly OT theories in mental health and provide the reader with references for further study. In the following, the approaches used in the various practices described throughout the book will be discussed in relation to the above-mentioned OT theories.

The practices described in the book can be organized into three major groups in relation to the knowledge base utilized.

Group One

This group consists of those who apply OTs philosophical principles directly to practice without defining explicitly a scientific theory and mostly work in directive relationships between symptoms or behaviours and activities. These include Chapters 2, 3, 4 and 6 which deal with the treatment of the long-term mentally ill in hospitals or in the community; OT in general hospitals or in day-treatment; and in the transition of chronic patients to independent living in the community. All four chapters discuss adult psychiatric patients in general terms. Chapters 2 and 6 discuss rehabilitation opportunities for long-term patients, whilst Chapters 3 and 4 discuss OT with acute as well as chronic patients also in short-term interventions. It can be said that these populations could be treated according to almost all of OT's theoretical approaches with appropriate modifications. They should benefit from Allen's cognitive theory which provides a measure of functional level and a task analysis procedure to guide treatment of chronic patients. Fidler's (1984) rehabilitation approach would be important to consider. The human occupation model could be utilized as well as Mosey's acquisitional or developmental frames of reference. King's application of sensory integration for chronic schizophrenics may contribute an additional perspective in this population.

The main point to stress here is the importance of using a conceptual model in clinical practice which guides systematic evaluation, intervention and research.

Group Two

This group presents practices which work also on the basis of OT philosophical principles, but in accordance with theories outside OT which are directly applied to practice. For example, behaviour modification in Chapters 6, 8, 13 and 16, which describe OT interventions with specially defined populations such as autistic children (Chapter 6), adolescents with conduct discorders (Chapter 8), head injuries (Chapter 13) and anorexia or bulimia nervosa (Chapter 16). In this group all ages are included, and all require long-term intervention in in-patient facilities.

Psychodynamic approaches in Chapters 6, 12 and 16 are another example of such applications, and although OT developed unique transformations of this knowledge base (Table 1.1), these are not used. In this category we may include also chapters which present mainly methods or techniques taken from other fields such as Chapter 10 on relaxation techniques, Chapter 6 on play and family therapy and Chapter 12 on psychodrama mentioned above.

Let us start by saying that preferably OT models should be employed. Thus, for example, behaviour modification techniques in general could be incorporated within an acquisitional frame of reference, or in combination with another model such as occupational behaviour as in Chapter 11. More specifically, regarding autistic children (Chapter 6), the literature on neuropsychological factors suggests that these factors probably contribute to the etiology of autism as Clarke (1983) summarizes. Therefore, in OT sensory integrative procedures may be beneficial for these children (Ayers, 1979; Ayers and Tickle, 1980; Clarke, 1983; Nelson, 1984; Peterson, 1986). Neuropathophysiological findings regarding the syndrome of autism have important implications for effective treatment as emphasized by Clarke (1983) and, hence, should be considered in OT.

With regard to eating disorders discussed in Chapter 16, two recent issues, one in *Occupational Therapy in Mental Health* (6, 1, 1986) and one in *Occupational Therapy in Health Care* (3, 2, 1986), are devoted to this subject. Most of these works in mental health utilize behavioural, cognitive-behavioural or the human occupational model, and also use activity groups.

Regarding head injuries (Chapter 13), a cognitive approach based on neuropsychology (Najenson *et al.*, 1984; Erickson, 1986; Averbuch and Katz, in press) in combination with Allen's theory, and in accordance with Luria's approach described in the chapter, could also be utilized. In addition, a cognitive group treatment can be based on Mosey's activities groups and developmental frame of reference as presented by Lundgren and Persechino (1986).

Group Three

This group consists of clinical practices which are based on OT philosophical principles and according to defined OT theories, such as Chapters 7, 9, 11, 14 and 15. Still, large differences exist among these in the comprehensiveness and adherence to a certain theory. The model of human occupation is used in Chapter 7 dealing with pediatric OT in integration with developmental perspectives. This model is also utilized in Chapter 14 in forensic psychiatry, and is mentioned in Chapter 11 on social skills training together with behaviour modification methods. In Chapter 15 on substance abuse Mosey's acquisitional frame of reference is mentioned together with Fidler's concepts of doing although what is described is not a fully systematic approach. Regarding OT in forensic psychiatry and substance abuse, Allen's cognitive approach would be beneficial and seems in accordance with the practice described; namely, sequencing steps in work according to capabilities and success (Chapter 14), or using structured task projects according to cognitive levels which are used also to reorganize rehabilitation activity groups (Chapter 15). In this case also biofeedback and relaxation techniques may be combined for stress management with OT concepts. These techniques which are presented in Chapter 10 have to be carefully considered as they are integrated in OT intervention.

Finally, Chapter 9 on groups provides a comprehensive review of OT literature related to groups, including Fidler's task oriented groups, Mosey's activities groups and Howe and Schwartzberg's functional groups (see Chapter 9 for references). Activity groups are among OT's legitimate tools (Mosey, 1981, 1986) and are part of almost all of the profession's frames of reference as outlined by Bruce. Regarding Allen's cognitive approach a detailed description of task groups according to cognitive levels is provided by Erdhardt in Allen (1985), which I, personally, would rather exclude under cognitive theory which is not necessarily developmental when concerned with adults.

In general, the choice of a theoretical approach and practical methods used by therapists are determined by the problem areas of the patient, the characteristics of the population, the age of the patient, the setting in which the intervention takes place, and the therapist's beliefs and expertise. As we may see from the above three groupings, none of these elements seems to determine the use or disuse of an OT theory in these practices. It is assumed that unfamiliarity with OT theories is among the reasons explaining the situation, hence the short literature review and references given here.

Concluding this section related to the science of OT, research activities in OT have to be mentioned. Diane Gibson, the editor of *Occupational Therapy Journal of Research,* wrote a compelling article on 'The dearth of mental health research in OT' (1984), in which she stresses the need for research based on theoretical frameworks to substantiate our effectiveness in practice. More recently, in *Occupational Therapy in Education: Target 2000* (1986), many leading figures in the profession emphasized that linking theory, research and practice is essential for the survival of the profession. Moreover, internalizing values and attitudes towards knowledge development is presented as central and critical for the future of OT and its credibility among the health professions.

As this book was not intended to focus on theoretical frameworks, but rather on practical issues, research findings are not presented in most chapters. It should, however, be emphasized again that without theory which guides practice and research no further growth is possible. In Chapter 13 on head injury rehabilitation, Giles presents findings from single subject research to demonstrate the effectiveness of treatment in specific cases. This method of research is advocated recently by Ottenbacher (1986) and Ottenbacher and Bonder (1986) as the most appropriate and feasible method for clinical research combining descriptions of individual cases with quantitative methods of analysis. This method of research should not be the only one, but it provides practitioners with one more way to study their evaluation and treatment procedures.

Domain of Concern, Aspects of Practice and Legitimate Tools: The Practice of OT

If we conceive philosophy as the 'why' OT is practising as it does, and theories guide 'what' or 'which' scientific data to use, the three additional elements of the professional model combined in this section are the 'where', 'when' and 'how' OT delivers its service. These are, in general terms, the areas of intervention, the sequence and focus of intervention and the methods how to intervene which are accepted by the profession and society at a certain time. These elements define what is included in practice but also what is excluded and do not belong. As the content of the model's elements changes over time these 'yeses' and 'nos' change also, but in any given time it seems to be important to remember that not everything is OT.

Domain of concern refers to the areas of OT's expertise consisting, according to Mosey (1981, 1986), of performance components and occupational performances within the context of age and environment. These components were reconsidered by Katz (1985) to consist of human occupation as the core within the context of competence components, age, cultural environment and time (see Figure 1.2). Using this perspective, OT practice can be analyzed in terms of what parts from the domain and in which manner were considered, in each individual case or in groups of individuals having something in common, and critically evaluate if other elements were necessary to consider as well.

The aspects of practice refer to the sequence and components of OT intervention. This includes, according to Mosey (1986), three major parts: evaluation, intervention, termination of treatment. Intervention is further subdivided into five types: meeting health needs, prevention, management, the change process, maintenance (p. 10). This sequence can be altered according to the case and the specific situation, as Mosey states, but it provides a way of organizing practice and evaluating it.

Legitimate tools of OT practice, according to Mosey, are '. . . the permissable means by which the practitioners of a profession fulfil their responsibility to society' (1986, p. 191). Mosey defines six general tools (not

Figure 1.2. Occupational Therapy Domain of Concern.

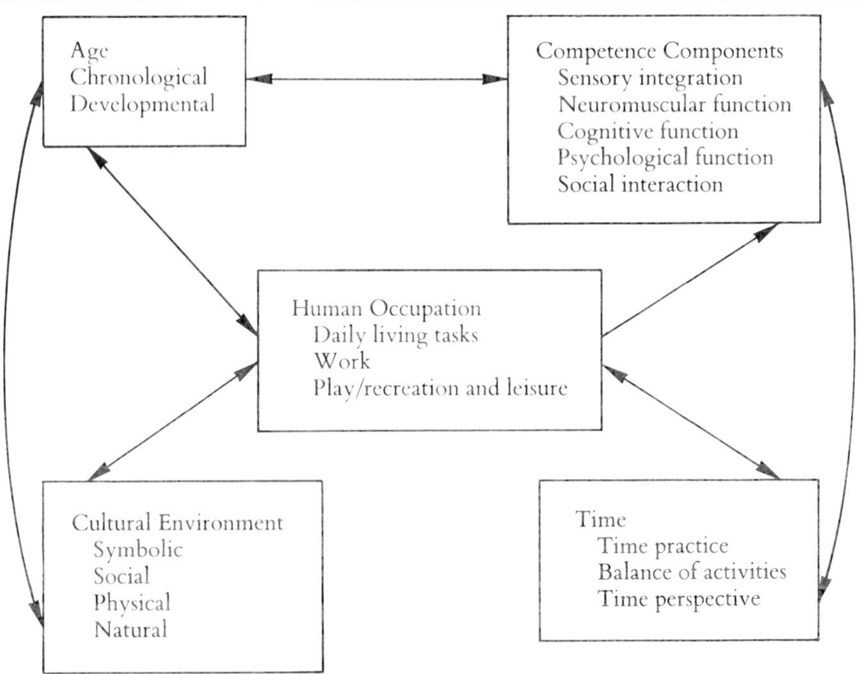

Reprinted with permission from the *American Occupational Therapy Journal*, Katz, 1985.

to be confused with specific examples of tools): non-human environment, conscious use of self, the teaching-learning process, purposeful activities, activity groups, activity analysis and synthesis. The focus is on OT's expertise in analyzing and adapting activities to be meaningful to the patient, in a teaching-learning process which may be individual or in groups, always involving the material environment and the resources of the therapist's self.

In summary, which of the components of each of the three elements outlined in this section are utilized by OTs in a specific case, are determined by the individual's problem areas, age and occupational history, but also by the frame of reference which guides therapists' practice and the setting in which they practice. This may explain the legitimate diversity in clinical practice so long as it is in accordance with the profession's philosophy and ethical codes.

Much consistency throughout the chapters of this book can be seen from the practising point of view, similar to the philosophical or art of therapy principles. All chapters deal with patients' occupational functions of daily tasks, work and recreation as the major focus. In addition, the competence components of psychological, cognitive and social interaction functions are the areas of interest (Figure 1.2). Age is considered when young populations are treated, but time factors and cultural environmental parameters are only rarely explicitly discussed. Konkol and Schneider in Chapter 15 on substance abuse and alcoholism use the domain model presented here including all its components in a population who suffer from mental as well as physical problems. As we deal in this book with mental health problems it is obvious that the same competence components are of concern, but the omission of time and environmental factors is crucial and these areas should be considered more in OT practice.

Among the aspects of OT practice, evaluation as the first step is mentioned in all chapters. In Chapter 3 examples of OT instruments are given, and a checklist for assessing problem areas is provided, although without relating this to the theories from which they derive, or suggesting a rationale 'when to use what'. In some chapters observation and interview are utilized. Reliable and valid assessment instruments in OT are essential, and therefore much research now centres on the development of instruments and the establishment of their measuring properties.

Following evaluation, the five intervention types suggested by Mosey for sequencing practice are not discussed with these terms in the book. But, if we take, for example, the intervention in head injury described by Giles in Chapter 13, in the first stages of recovery the focus is on 'meeting health needs', while in the second and third stages the 'change process' or 'maintenance' are the foci of the rehabilitation process. Prevention is mentioned, for example, in Chapter 3 from a counselling aspect, assisting in planning free time as a preventative measure, and 'management' is the focus in Chapter 8 where the treatment of conduct disorders is described. Termination of treatment is not explicitly defined in most chapters (excluding Chapters 14 and 15), reflecting one of OT's difficulties in clearly defining its contribution.

Occupational therapy practice in the past centred on treatment methods and modalities and neglected evaluation which enables systematic treatment planning, as well as determining the point of termination and follow-up. As mentioned above, this situation is changing and practitioners are advised to use evaluation instruments to guide all phases of practice.

Among OT legitimate tools, as defined by Mosey, activity groups is the one method mentioned in all chapters. It appears that this tool is useful for all populations, ages and settings with appropriate adaptations of size, media, environment and manners of leadership. Using material objects and providing purposeful activity seem embedded in the principles of practice, while the other tools, as Mosey defines them, are mentioned only in a few cases like the process of teaching-learning in Chapter 5; conscious use of self is part of the psychodynamic approaches in Chapters 6 and 12; and activity analysis is mentioned in Chapters 9 and 11. Among these, activity analysis is crucial for OT practice and is a major expertise of the profession's, thus methods of activity analysis have to be utilized and presented as part of OT's clinical work (Fidler, 1963; Tiffany, 1983; Allen, 1985; Kielhofner, 1985; Mosey, 1986).

Conclusion

Occupational therapy's philosophical principles appear as the unifying elements of the profession in the clinical applications presented in this book. Namely, the art of therapy is the most stable and accepted basis for OT practice. On the other hand, OT's diversity should result not only because patient populations vary and settings are different, but also because different theoretical models are utilized to guide practice and research, so that practitioners can choose in accordance with their beliefs and values, from an array of models and theories, the appropriate one for the individual patient or the specific population of interest.

The purpose here was to enhance the utilization of theoretical models in OT practice by providing a conceptual perspective to analyze practice, and to direct readers to references taken from OT literature. I am sure that all we contributors to this book see our work as ever-changing and developing towards a more systematic and effective service to our patients and society.

References

ALLEN, C.K. (1982) 'Independence through activity: The practice of occupational therapy (psychiatry)', *American Journal of Occupational Therapy,* 36, 731–9.

ALLEN, C.K. (1985) *Occupational Therapy for Psychiatric Diseases: Measurement and Management of Cognitive Disabilities.* Boston, Mass., Little Brown.

ALLEN, C.K. (1987) 'Activity: Occupational therapy's treatment method', *Eleanor Clarke Slagle Lectureship,* presented at the AOTA Conference, Indianapolis.

AVERBURCH, S. and Katz, N. (in press) 'Assessment of perceptual cognitive performance of psychiatric and brain injured adult patients', *Occupational Therapy in Mental Health,* 8.

AYERS, A.J. (1972) *Sensory Integration and Learning Disorders,* Los Angeles, Calif., Western Psychological Services.

AYERS, A.J. (1979) *Sensory Integration and the Child,* Los Angeles, Calif., Western Psychological Services.

AYERS, A.J. and TICKLE, L.S. (1980) 'Hyperresponsivity to touch and vestibular stimulation as a predictor of positive response to sensory integration procedures by autistic children', *American Journal of Occupational Therapy,* 34, 375–81.

AZIMA, H. and AZIMA, F. (1959) 'Outline of a dynamic theory of occupational therapy', *American Journal of Occupational Therapy,* 13, 215–19.

BARRIS, R., KIELHOFNER, G. and WATTS, J.H. (1983) *Psychosocial Occupational Therapy,* Laural, Md., Ramsco Publishing.

BAUM, C.M. (1980) 'Occupational therapists put care in the health system', *American Journal of Occupational Therapy,* 34, 505–16.

BING, R.K. (1981) 'Occupational therapy revisited: A paraphrastic journey', Eleanor Clarke Sagle Lectureship, *American Journal of Occupational Therapy,* 35, 499–518.

BING, R.K. (1986) 'Perspectives on the values underlying occupational therapy practice', in *Occupational Therapy Education Target 2000 Proceedings,* The American Occupational Therapy Association, p. 215.

BRIGGS, A.K., DUNSCOMBE, L.W., HOWE, M.C. and SCHWARTZBERG, S.L. (1979) *Case Simulations in Psychosocial Occupational Therapy,* Philadelphia, Penn., F.A. Davis.

BURKE, J.P. (1977) 'A clinical perspective on motivation: Pawn versus origin,' *American Journal of Occupational Therapy,* 31, 254–8.

CLARK, F. (1983) 'Research on the neuropathophysiology of autism and its implications for occupational therapy', *The Occupational Therapy Journal of Research,* 3, 3–22.

CLARKE, P.N. (1979) 'Human development through occupation: Theoretical frameworks in contemporary occupational therapy, Part 1', *American Journal of Occupational Therapy,* 33, 505–14.

DENTON, P.L. (1987) *Psychiatric Occupational Therapy: A Workbook of Practical Skills,* Boston, Mass., Little Brown.

DUNNING, R.E. (1973) 'Philosophy and occupational therapy', *American Journal of Occupational Therapy,* 27, 18–23.

ENGELHARDT, H.T. (1977) 'Defining occupational therapy', *American Journal of Occupational Therapy,* 27, 18–23.

ENGELHARDT, H.T. (1986) 'The importance of values in shaping professional direction and behaviour', in *Occupational Therapy Education Target 2000 Proceedings,* The American Occupational Therapy Association, pp. 39–43.

ERICKSON, B.C. (1986) 'In search of brain-behaviour relationships in dementia and the Luria-Nebraska neuropsychological battery,' *Physical and Occupational Therapy in Geriatrics,* 4, 113–39.

FIDLER, G.S. (1981) 'From crafts to competence', *American Journal of Occupational Therapy,* 35, 567–73.

FIDLER, G.S. (1982) 'The Lifestyle Performance Profile: An organizing frame', in B.J. HEMPHILL (Ed.), *The Evaluative Process in Occupational Therapy.* Thorofare, N.J., Charles B. Slack, pp 43–7.

FIDLER, G.S. (1984) *Design of Rehabilitation Services in Psychiatric Hospital Settings',* Laural, Md., Ramsco Publishing.

FIDLER, G.S. and FIDLER, J.W. (1954) *Introduction to Psychiatric Occupational Therapy,* New York, Harper and Row.

FIDLER, G.S. and FIDLER, J.W. (1963) *Occupational Therapy: A Communication Process in Psychiatry,* New York, Macmillan.

FIDLER, G.S. and FIDLER, J.W. (1978) 'Doing and becoming: Purposeful action and self-actualization', *American Journal of Occupational Therapy,* 32, 305–10.

GIBSON, D. (1984) 'The dearth of mental health research in occupational therapy', *The Occupational Therapy Journal of Research',* 4, 131–49.

GILFOYLE,, E.M. (1980) 'Caring: A philosophy for practice', *American Journal of Occupational Therapy,* 34, 517–21.

HEMPHILL, B.J. (1982) *The Evaluative Process in Psychiatric Occupational Therapy,* Thorofare, N.J., Charles B. Slack.

JOHNSON, J.A. (1977) 'Humanitarianism and accountability: A challenge for occupational therapy on its 60th anniversary', *American Journal of Occupational Therapy,* 31, 631–7.

KATZ, N. (1985) 'Occupational therapy's domain of concern: Reconsidered', *American Journal of Occupational Therapy,* 39, 518–24.

KATZ, N., JOSMAN, N. and STEINMEZ, N. (in press) 'Relationship between cognitive disability theory and the human occupation model in the assessment of psychiatric and non-psychiatric adolescents', *Occupational Therapy in Mental Health,* 8.

KIELHOFNER, G. (1980a) 'A model of human occupation. Part 2: Ontogenesis from the perspective of temporal adaptation', *American Journal of Occupational Therapy,* 34, 657–63.

KIELHOFNER, G. (1980b) 'A model of human occupation. Part 3: Benign and vicious cycles', *American Journal of Occupational Therapy,* 34, 731–7.

KIELHOFNER, G. (1983) *Health through Occupation: Theory and Practice in Occupational Therapy,* Philadelphia, Pa., F.A. Davis.

KIELHOFNER, G. (1985) *A Model of Human Occupation,* Baltimore, Md., Williams and Wilkins.

KIELHOFNER, G. and BURKE, J. (1980) 'A model of human occupation. Part 1: Conceptual framework and content', *American Journal of Occupational Therapy,* 34, 571–81.

KIELHOFNER, G., BURKE, J. and IGI, C. (1980) 'A model of human occupation. Part 4: Assessment and intervention', *American Journal of Occupational Therapy,* 34, 777–88.

KING, L.J. (1974) 'A sensory integrative approach to schizophrenia', *American Journal of Occupational Therapy,* 28, 529–36.

KING, L.J. (1978) 'Eleanor Clarke Slagle lectureship: Towards a science of adaptive responses', *American Journal of occupational Therapy,* 32, 429–37.

KING, L.J. (1980) 'Creative caring', *American Journal of Occupational Therapy,* 34, 522–8.

KING, L.J. (1982) 'The Person Symbol as an assessment tool', in B.J. HEMPHILL (Ed.), *The Evaluative Process in Psychiatric Occupational Therapy,* Thorofare, N.J., Charles B. Slack, pp. 169–94.

KREFTING, L.H. (1985) 'The use of conceptual models in clinical practice', *Canadian Journal of Occupational Therapy,* 52, 173–8.

LEVY, L.L. (1987) 'Psychosocial interventions and dementia, Part 1: State of the art, future directions', *Occupational Therapy in Mental Health,* 7, 69–107.

LLORENS, L.A. (1970a) '1969 Eleanor Clarke Slagle Lectureship: Facilitating growth and development: The promise of occupational therapy', *American Journal of Occupational Therapy,* 24, 1–9.

LLORENS, L.A. (1970b) 'Application of a developmental theory for health and rehabilitation', Rockville, Md., American Occupational Therapy Association.

LLORENS, L.A. (1984) 'Theoretical conceptualizations of occupational therapy', *Occupational Therapy in Mental Health,* 4, 1–14.

LUNDGREN, C.C. and PERSECHINO, E.L. (1986) 'Cognitive group: A treatment program for head injured adults', *American Journal of Occupational Therapy,* 40, 397–401.

MAYER, M.A. 'Analysis of information processing and cognitive disability theory', *American Journal of Occupational Therapy,* 42, 3, 176–183.

MEYER, M.A. (1977) 'The philosophy of occupational therapy', *American Journal of Occupational Therapy,* 31, 639–42.

MOSEY, A.C. (1970) *Three Frames of Reference for Mental Health,* Thorofare, N.J., Charles B. Slack.

MOSEY, A.C. (1973) *Activities Therapy,* New York, Raven Press.

MOSEY, A.C. (01981) *Occupational Therapy: Configuration of a Profession,* New York, Raven Press.

MOSEY, A.C. (1985) 'A monistic or a pluralistic approach to professional identity', *American Journal of Occupational Therapy,* 39, 504–9.

MOSEY, A.C. (1986) *Psychosocial Components of Occupational Therapy,* New York, Raven Press.

NAJENSON, T., RAHMANI, L., ELASAR, B. and AVERBUCH, S. (1984) 'An elementary cognitive assessment and treatment of the craniocerebrally injured patient', in EDELSTEIN, B.A. and COUTURE, E.T. (Eds), *Behavioural Assessment and Rehabilitation of the Traumatically Brain-damaged,* New York, Plenum Press, pp. 313–38.

NELSON, D.L. (1984) *Children with Autism and Other Pervasive Disorders of Development and Behaviour: Therapy through Activities,* Thorofare, N.J., Charles B. Slack.

OTTENBACHER, K.J. (1986) *Evaluating Clinical Change: Strategies for Occupational and Physical Therapists,* Baltimore, Md., Williams and Wilkins.

OTTENBACHER, K.J. and BONDER, B.B. (1986) *Scientific Inquiry: Design and Analysis Issues in Occupational Therapy,* Rockville, Md., American Occupational Therapy Association.

OWEN, G.M. (1968) 'An analysis of the philosophy of occupational therapy', *American Journal of Occupational Therapy,* 22, 502–5.

PARUSH, S., LAPIDOT, G., EDELSTEIN, P.V and TAMIR, D. (1987)'Occupational therapy in mother and child health care centers', *American Journal of Occupational Therapy*, 31, 9, 601–605.

PETERSON, T.W. (1986) 'Recent studies in autism: A review of the literature', *Occupational Therapy in Mental Health*, 6, 63–75.

REED, K.L. (1984) *Models of Practice in Occupational Therapy*, Baltimore, Md., Williams and Wilkins.

REILLY, M. (1966) 'A psychiatric occupational therapy program as a teaching model', *American Journal of Occupational Therapy*, 20, 61–7.

REILLY, M. (1969) 'The education process', *American Journal of Occupational Therapy*, 23, 300–3.

REILLY, M. (1974) *Play as Exploratory Learning*, Beverley Hills, Calif., Sage Publications.

REYNOLDS, P.D. (1971) *A Primer in Theory Construction*, Indianapolis, Ind., Bobbs-Merrill.

ROSS, M. and BURDICK, D. (1981) *Sensory Integration*, Thorofare, N.J., Charles B. Slack.

SCHROEDER, C.V., BLOCK, M.P. TROTTIER, E.C. and STOWELL, M.S. (1982) 'The adult psychiatric sensory integration evaluation, in HEMPHILL, B.J. (Ed.), *The Evaluative Process in Psychiatric Occupational Therapy*, Thorofare, N.J., Charles B. Slack, pp. 227–53.

SIEG, K.W. (1974) 'Applying the behavioural model to the occupational therapy model', *American Journal of Occupational Therapy*, 28, 421–8.

TIFFANY, E.G. (1983) 'Psychiatry and mental health', in HOPKINS, H.L. and SMITH, H.D. (Eds), *Willard and Spackman's Occupational Therapy*, 6th ed., Philadelphia, Pa., J.B. Lippincott, Ch. 19.

WILSON, M. (1983) *Occupational Therapy in Long Term Psychiatry*, New York, Churchill Livingstone.

YERXA, E.B. (1967) 'Authentic occupational therapy', The Eleanor Clark Slagle Lectureship, *American Journal of Occupational Therapy*, 21, 155–73.

YERXA, E.B. (1980) 'Occupational therapy's role in creating a future climate of caring', *American Journal of Occupational Therapy*, 34, 529–34.

YERXA, E.B. (1983) 'Audacious values: The energy source for occupational therapy', in G. Kielhofner (Ed.), *Health through Occupation: Theory and Practice in Occupational Therapy*, Philadelphia, Pa., F.A. Davis, pp. 149–62.

Chapter 2

Treatment of the Long-Term Mentally Ill

Terry Krupa, Marge Murphy and John Thornton

Recently much attention has been focused on the dilemma of the long-term psychiatric population (Anthony, 1979; Stern and Minkoff, 1979; Lamb, 1982). There has been a resurgence of interest in the nature of long-term mental illness and the development of strategies to promote recovery, optimal functioning and quality of life. From its earliest days OT has recognized the profession's involvement with this group (Bing, 1981). The principles and philosophies embodied in OT readily lend themselves to making a valuable contribution in the area of long-term mental illness. This chapter looks at a variety of theoretical and practical issues facing OTs working in this field. Although the challenges and difficulties are frankly presented, the intentions are to stimulate OTs' involvement in a satisfying and rewarding area of practice.

While OTs begin their involvement with the client during the period of acute symptomatology, the majority of their efforts will take place once the positive symptoms (e.g., delusions) are stabilized and the negative symptoms (e.g., social withdrawal) are the most prominent impairments.

Skills and Resource Deficits

A variety of skill and resource deficits may disturb the ability of the long-term mentally ill's to function in a satisfying and effective manner in their living, learning, working and social environments. Skill deficits can include physical skills (e.g., stamina, strength, coordination), emotional skills (making and maintaining friendships, dealing with interpersonal conflicts, maintaining commitments, cooperation) and intellectual skills (e.g., memory, concentration, problem-solving).

Unfortunately, the resources required for the rehabilitation of this population are frequently limited or unsatisfactory. Resources required include material goods (e.g., clothing, furniture, finances, housing), places (e.g., social clubs, employment agencies, housing options), or social resources to provide support, friendship and caring relationships (e.g., family, friends, colleagues) (Anthony, 1979; Anthony *et al.*, 1978).

Psychological Issues and Social Issues

It is not surprising that long-term mental illness interferes with an individual's psychological well-being. Self-esteem, self-confidence and the ability to hope for a satisfying and meaningful future are all affected. Furthermore, society typically demonstrates a poor understanding and even less sympathy for those affected by psychiatric disabilities. Myths about mental illness and the social stigma handicap an individual's ability to develop an integrated, meaningful and satisfying lifestyle (Anthony and Liberman, 1986; Strauss, 1986).

Case Profile

To illustrate these difficulties and how they impact on OT the following case example is presented. 'Peter' is a 30-year-old single male. He has a primary psychiatric diagnosis of chronic schizophrenia, and a secondary diagnosis of personality disorder. He has required several inpatient hospitalizations over the past eight years, usually because of an exacerbation of his acute psychiatric symptoms. These acute symptoms include auditory hallucinations, delusions of musical fame and the belief that he has the ability to influence musicians. These symptoms are usually controlled with injectable neuroleptic medications. Peter, however, does not acknowledge his symptoms as illness and is subsequently unreliable with respect to medications. When the acute symptoms are controlled, Peter presents as apathetic and lacking in direction, low in energy, affectively flat and socially isolated. His personal grooming is poor and his clothing ill-fitting and untidy.

Peter's family includes his mother and father who are divorced but living in the same city. Both are employed. His 19-year-old brother attends university. Peter has no contact with his father or brother. He speaks to his mother weekly by telephone and visits her only upon her invitation. Mother feels Peter should be directed towards university level studies in the future.

Peter shares a room with three other residents in a minimally supervised boarding home, located in a poor socioeconomic district of a large city. He completed grade 12 and the first half-year of a university electrical engineering course. Attempts to return to university were foiled by a return of acute symptoms, and his inability to meet the emotional and intellectual demands of the course. His work history has been limited and transient in nature. He receives a disability income which barely covers his basic monthly expenses. He views his part-time work assembling electrical equipment at a sheltered workshop as preparation for a career in the electronics field.

Socially, he spends much time alone and wishes he had kept in contact with his old school acquaintances. He drinks large amounts of coffee and smokes thirty-five cigarettes per day. Occasionally he likes to repair small electrical appliances. He attends a drop-in centre for ex-psychiatric patients once a week.

Defining a Focus for Occupational Therapy

The long-term mentally ill have a broad spectrum of needs which require attention. Having identified a specific need, the OT must also consider how it relates to other aspects of the client's situation. In our case example the OT should not approach Peter's lack of recreational pursuits separately from his financial situation. Peter's desire to return to a university level electronics career appears straightforward on the surface. However, it is a poorly thought out attempt to regain self-respect and define a meaningful future. This is being reinforced by his past educational experiences, his brother's status as a university student, and his mother's expectation for his academic future.

Maintaining a holistic perspective also ensures that the OT is aware of the many different, but complementary, treatment approaches which may be required by the long-term mentally ill. Medical management, pharmacotherapy, crisis intervention, health education, family therapy, psychotherapy and rehabilitation are only a sample of the comprehensive array of treatment approaches which must be coordinated.

OTs must also be clear about how they can contribute to the treatment process; that is, the roles, knowledge and skills the profession identifies as its areas of expertise. For OT the areas of work, play and self-care are the focus. OTs help their clients to achieve effective and satisfying performance in these areas (Barris *et al.*, 1983). It requires a specialist level of knowledge and skill to be able to understand and remediate those factors that may lead to dysfunction. While the OT may have some knowledge and skill in treatment areas which fall outside the domain of OT, at times it may be most appropriate for a specialist from another discipline to become involved.

Management Principles for Occupational Therapy

Facilitating Client Involvement

Client involvement helps to ensure interest, acceptance and participation in the OT programme and promotes the development of independence in satisfying and effective occupational performance. Client involvement can be particularly difficult to achieve with the long-term mentally ill who possess a multitude of disabilities that leave them marginal or passive participants in many aspects of life.

Client involvement begins during assessment, the initial stage of OT. The assessment provides the therapist with a baseline of information to develop a programme based on the client's strengths and deficits. If there is a lack of agreement between the client and therapist with respect to the process and the results of the assessment, then client involvement in developing goals and programme plans is compromised.

To facilitate client involvement the therapist must be prepared to orient the long-term mentally ill client to the components of the assessment process and their relevance. Education about the nature of the dysfunction is important. Orientation and education helps clarify and personalize the process for the client. Subsequently the client may also be more amenable to addressing issues which are particularly threatening (e.g., mental illness, personal competence, unrealistic goals, limited supports).

The assessment should highlight those aspects of the client's occupational performance which remain intact and incorporate them as much as possible into the OT goals and plans. This may be particularly difficult with the long-term mentally ill who appear to have so few strengths, uneven performance abilities and are subject to so many environments that are not empathetic, flexible or accommodating. Yet the creative therapist who respects the client's strengths will attempt to translate them into a manageable and meaningful programme of activities and likely enhance client involvement. Had the therapist working with Peter been overwhelmed by his needs and deficits, then his interest in electronics might have been ignored, or perceived as a negative, unrealistic factor. Instead, the therapist used his interest constructively to negotiate an appealing and therapeutic programme of activities.

Facilitating Motivation

Disturbances of motivation are frequent among the long-term mentally ill. The outward presentation of motivational difficulties may include a dull and blunted affect, apathy, social withdrawal, limited participation in goal-oriented activity and a lack of self-direction. These disturbances in motivation are particularly troublesome because they appear to be intrinsic. That is, these individuals often appear disinterested in activity for the personal rewards of achievement and mastery. The result is a withdrawal from activity, both task-oriented and interpersonal, and a subsequent deterioration of skills and resources. The psychological effects include a loss of self-esteem and self-confidence and a disturbed sense of personal effectiveness, which all perpetuate a cycle of inactivity (Liberman *et al.*, 1982).

Given the overwhelming impact of their psychiatric difficulties on their personal lives, it is understandable that many clients present with poorly developed goals, values, interests and pleasures. Also these motivational disturbances and their outward presentations make it difficult for the OT to establish a therapeutic relationship. The therapist must develop a therapeutic relationship with the client based on the assumption that motivational disturbances do not reflect a total absence of motivation. These individuals all have interests, values, pleasures and preferences which they are often unaware of, that can be developed and result in an increase in their involvement in activity.

Establishing the therapeutic relationship is the first step in facilitating motivation. While these individuals may tax any unexpecting therapist's ability to develop a therapeutic relationship, it can be achieved with time, patience and a willingness to listen and appreciate the client's unique needs and strengths. The purpose of the therapeutic relationship is to:

1 develop a safe, supportive and accepting relationship where the client can feel free to explore potential sources of internal motivation (e.g., interests, values, pleasures, preferences) without fear of reprisal, judgment or failure;
2 help the client gain greater self-understanding through feeling understood;
3 help the person hope again through recognizing his potential to achieve and to be more self-directed;
4 develop the role of mediator where the individual can draw on the therapist's intact energy, drive, skills, perceptions, judgments, etc. when required;
5 develop with their therapist rehabilitation goals, plans and actions (Anthony, 1980; Keats and McGlashan, 1985).

By exploring the client's internal sources of motivation both therapist and client are in a better position to develop manageable and reasonable rehabilitation goals and plans. This is an ongoing process and cannot be rushed as the level and nature of the client's involvement in activities will change with new experiences, and the development of the client's skills and resources (Krupa and Thornton, 1986). In our example Peter participated only in passive and solitary leisure activities when first introduced to his OT. Through their relationship they became aware of his interest in electronics and his high regard for education, and identified those factors that would interfere with these goals. With his OT Peter was able to set a manageable short-term goal of part-time sheltered employment with exposure to electronics assembly. While electronics study is a long-term goal, Peter finds many aspects of the workshop experience meaningful and satisfying.

Developing Personal Skills

The value of skill training with the long-term mentally ill has been widely acknowledged (Wallace *et al.*, 1980; Liberman *et al.*, 1985). The goal of developing personal skills by OT is to improve the individual's competency for coping in an effective and satisfying manner with the demands of everyday living. Skill development will be most useful and meaningful if the skills to be developed are consistent with the client's interests, values and needs and are perceived as appropriate to the demands of the client's natural environments (Barris *et al.*, 1983). Peter, for example, was amenable to developing specific work skills on a sheltered workshop assembly line because he perceived them as related to at least some of the demands he could expect in an electronics job.

Skill training for the long-term mentally ill must be graded at several levels. First, the therapist must be concerned about the amount of activity and new learning for those clients who have led relatively unproductive lifestyles, or are recuperating from an acute relapse of their psychiatric symptoms. Too much activity too soon may overwhelm and demoralize. To avoid the client withdrawing from activity, and perhaps from the therapeutic relationship, the therapist must be sensitive to the client's tolerance for activity while ensuring continued interest and involvement (Krupa and Thornton, 1986).

The environment where skill development takes place must also be graded. While the hospital office or agency environment may be a safe and trustworthy place to learn and practise new skills, it does not guarantee that accomplishments will be generalized to other environments (Liberman *et al.*, 1986). Each environment has both obvious and subtle differences in the demands placed on the individual's personal skills. The demands of an employment programme will, for example, require many skills of Peter that he has not been expected to develop in the sheltered workshop. The OT programme must provide opportunities for the client to apply newly learned skills in all of the appropriate environments.

Finally, the OT must grade the nature of reinforcements provided to support the client's efforts in skill development. Reinforcements are particularly important for those individuals who have poorly developed systems of intrinsic motivation as they are less likely to participate in new learning for the pleasures of achievement and mastery. The OT must be creative in the search for reinforcers that are perceived by the clients as rewarding, and which can be carried into the client's natural environments (Brown, 1982; Liberman, 1982; Liberman *et al.*, 1982). This may require the therapist to begin with external reinforcers (e.g., money, praise, special privileges) to involve the client in successful activities, and eventually to shape the client's responses to a point where intrinsic reinforcements can become effective motivators.

Developing Resources

The OT working with the long-term mentally ill must be prepared to intervene when factors external to the client promote or maintain dysfunction. The goal is to modify existing environments, and to develop new resources to facilitate the client's satisfactory community adjustment (Anthony and Liberman, 1986). All people require, at the very minimum, the resources to meet basic survival needs (food, shelter, clothing). For the long-term mentally ill who are generally dependent on social programmes or family members, meeting basic survival needs may stretch their resources to the limit. Those individuals with long-term psychiatric disabilities will require new and expanded resources if they are to be successful. While the OT may provide the client with the opportunities and experiences for rehabilitation, the OT must also ensure the presence of needed resources by teaching, negotiating and advocating on the client's behalf. For Peter the OT needed to negotiate extra transportation funds with the relevant authorities to facilitate his attendance at the sheltered workshop programme. The therapist also worked with the client's mother, workshop counsellor and workshop supervisors to provide the level and nature of support needed to ensure Peter's progress in the vocational rehabilitation programme.

Measuring Outcomes

OTs have become increasingly aware of the need to demonstrate the effectiveness of their services. The issues of economic restraint, quality assurance and professional accountability have made evaluation an essential component of any OT service. Developing sound and rigorous methods for evaluation can be particularly problematic for therapists working with the long-term mentally ill. As Peter's case demonstrates, these clients typically present with a wide variety of difficulties of interest to the OT. Within each of these areas the OT must define observable and measurable variables. While this is a difficult task for specific skill or resource development, it becomes especially problematic to define the measurements for such vague and subjective variables as 'self-esteem' and 'self-confidence'. Furthermore, therapists must determine suitable units of measurement without losing any sense of comprehensiveness and relevance (Anthony and Farkas, 1982). In the case of Peter it would be difficult to appreciate the benefits of OT intervention if outcome measures were to focus on only small units of social development (e.g., bowling weekly or completing an electronics project). The OT must identify a range of measurable units that will provide a meaningful picture of the individual's psychosocial development.

Remember that even if all of the client's strengths, limitations and needs were identified in measurable units and an OT programme developed, it would still be difficult to establish conclusively the cause of any changes or improvements (Kanter, 1985). Bachrach (1982) points out that even modest goals may be the result of a number of different variables or their interactive effects. Peter was involved in several different treatment approaches. Rehabilitation efforts were often accompanied by crisis management and drug therapy. Furthermore, besides OT Peter had involvement with other professionals, peers and family members 'each with its own particular set of standards and intervention capabilities' (Malm *et al.*, 1981). Similarly, social and financial policies and the labour market reflect only some of the influences of the larger society. While it is important that the OT be aware of these confounding variables and their potential effects, it is impossible and often unethical to control them. To withhold certain treatments from Peter in order to see the effects of OT interventions in a purer form would not be reasonable.

In addition, OTs must look beyond the presence or absence of a predicted change. Liberman (1982) suggests a multi-level approach for assessing treatment outcomes. First, Liberman states that skills should be evaluated according to their generalization into new and natural settings. The OT working with Peter would ensure that the skills of personal grooming he has learned in a life skills group are carried out at his boarding home. Secondly, there is the question of durability. How long do these new skills last with and without support? Does Peter maintain these skills over time, or does he stop performing them shortly after the group is ended? Finally, do any of these skills held reduce symptoms or improve psychosocial functioning? Is Peter's presence more easily accepted at his mother's home and in local coffee shops?

The concept of outcome measurement also implies a comparison of criteria pre- and post-treatment. Yet Peter's lengthy psychiatric history illustrates that the possibilities for 'concluding' occupational treatment with the long-term mentally ill are questionable. The changes made with this population usually take time, and fluctuations in the client's psychiatric and psychosocial functioning may disrupt the progress that has been achieved. Liberman (1982) suggests that positive treatment results with the long-term mentally ill are only likely to occur within the context of a relationship lasting a minimum of six months and up to four years.

The OT working with Peter is fortunate to work within a programme that allows for the long-term commitment necessary to achieve gains in psychosocial functioning. The reality is that many OTs cannot remain actively involved beyond inpatient hospitalization, day programming or perhaps other time limited interventions. These therapists must establish their outcome measurements accordingly.

Defining Success

Relapse and post-hospital employment are the traditional measures of success in psychiatric rehabilitation (Anthony, 1979; Anthony *et al.*, 1978; Anthony and Farkas, 1982). If we were to use relapse and post-hospital employment as our measures of successful rehabilitation, then our case study would seem destined for failure. Recent studies have indicated that although the long-term mentally ill may share common diagnoses, they are all unique individuals with respect to their potential for rehabilitation (Anthony, 1979). Despite a diagnosis of schizophrenia, Peter differs from other clients in the details of his background history, vocational, social, and personality characteristics and his available skills and resources. A difficulty in the treatment of the long-term mentally ill is that it is essentially impossible objectively to generalize the prediction of outcomes (Anthony *et al.*, 1978). One can only define what can be reasonably expected from any one client.

The issue of success is further complicated by characteristic fluctuations of functional level. As Peter demonstrates, the OT must motivate the withdrawn, underactive and apathetic client. Yet relapse of acute symptomatology may be exacerbated if the client is overstimulated or pressured by demanding environments. In his writings on the long-term mentally ill, Lamb (1982) stresses that despite this precarious situation, therapists should assist the client to the highest level of functional independence while maintaining a realistic perspective on the individual's potential for rehabilitation. The therapist must be aware of how much activity to introduce while maintaining the client's involvement and ensuring a course of rehabilitation progress. It is important for the therapist to recognize that brief relapses of acute symptomatology can occur within a context of psychosocial improvement. OTs must maintain a flexible perspective on success. If we were to consider Peter's most recent admission to hospital as a failure, we would be overlooking his general gains in psychosocial functioning. While he may not be pursuing the academic studies he desires, he has been able to invest in a vocational programme with some specific rehabilitation goals in mind. Even a return to hospital does not have to negate achievements made by Peter, and the skills and resources he has developed will potentially survive and facilitate his re-entry into the community.

Several studies have focused attention on the dangers inherent in models of rehabilitation that measure success by high levels of achievement. Lamb (1981, 1982) stresses that therapists who set goals beyond the client's ability are similar to therapists who avoid involvement with this group because they both promote failure and reaffirm the client's helplessness and chronic status. Furthermore, Lamb proposes that setting goals that can never be met will only serve to frustrate therapists and ultimately compromise the status of psychiatric rehabilitation. There is the danger that we may discredit the whole idea of rehabilitation if we oversell it and make promises we cannot keep (Lamb, 1982, p. 17). When this occurs, long-term clients are most vulnerable to neglect.

Perhaps the greatest danger with the traditional measures of success in psychiatric rehabilitation is that they do not address the fundamental issues of quality of life and the client's perceptions of what constitutes a satisfying and meaningful existence. Fine (1980) reminds us that 'outcome with the chronic population should not be measured with the same yardstick used for the acutely ill and less disabled' (p. 52).

Malm *et al.* (1981) point out that given the wide range of factors that are considered the responsibility of health care professionals, those features of life that are of personal importance to the client are at risk of being neglected, particularly when the wishes of the client are at odds with social standards. Even the values and interests of the OT can subtly influence the development of the rehabilitation plan. However, without Peter's involvement in this process the result is likely to be disinterest or resistance. Unfortunately, it is this type of situation that is frequently explained as the client's lack of motivation, or as a factor related to the illness process.

To summarize, OT interventions that are based on unrealistic assumptions regarding the rehabilitation process will likely prove unrewarding both to client and therapist. Success in the psychiatric rehabilitation of the long-term mentally ill can only be measured on an individual basis and with broad and flexible terms. It is the task of the OT to determine with the client not only where gains in psychosocial functioning are desired and required but also which specific gains can be realistically expected.

Maintaining Professional Interest

Stern and Minkoff (1979) elaborate on several 'paradoxes' leading to stress in working with the long-term mentally ill that can affect OTs. While realizing that many patients cannot be cured, therapists must justify their therapeutic efforts in a health system that historically gives low status to the rehabilitation of this group. Added to this, clients who are socially and emotionally unresponsive and progress slowly and minimally can facilitate a sense of futility and prove professionally unrewarding for the unprepared therapist.

This situation is magnified by social and economic factors that affect the rehabilitation process. Poor social support systems, social stigma, community intolerance, inflation and meagre financial assistance benefits, inadequate housing, unemployment and the changes in the technological and labour demands of the work force are all factors to contend with. All these issues raise the question: What are we rehabilitating our clients for?

Lamb (1982) delineates a final source of stress which is particularly relevant to psychiatric OTs. While many clients may refuse involvement in rehabilitation, this is especially common with the long-term mentally ill. Activity, the basis of the practice of OT, is considered an essential component in the development of personal competence and skills of mastery. The long-term mentally ill who reject therapeutic activity challenge the professional integrity of OT. For this reason Lamb stresses the importance for all professionals to examine their motivation and needs in working with the mentally ill.

Conclusion

From one perspective, working with the long-term mentally ill lacks the excitement of the acutely ill, the predictability of well defined illnesses, the immediate rewards of treating the less disabled and the appeal of the socially stable client. Yet for therapists who are willing to re-evaluate the needs and potentials of the long-term mentally ill there exists a meaningful and attractive philosophy for treatment.

As the interest in the rehabilitation needs of the long-term mentally ill grows, so does the demand for OT services. Therapists are required for this area of practice in traditional hospital settings and also in the community-based rehabilitation programmes that service this population. Furthermore, there is a need for innovative therapists willing to design and implement new interventions and participate in research efforts to demonstrate their effectiveness. Finally, the field of mental health, perhaps more than any other, requires the knowledge, experience and energy to meet the challenge of inappropriate social policies and inadequate resources. Occupational therapists with an interest in this area of mental health service delivery will be in step with the profession's direction for the twenty-first century.

Acknowledgment

Parts of this chapter are based on an article, 'Occupational therapy issues in the treatment of the long term mentally ill' by Terry Krupa, Connie Hayashi, Marge Murphy and John Thornton, published in the *Canadian Journal of Occupational Therapy*, 52, 3, 1985, 105–11, and are reproduced with permission.

References

ANTHONY, W. (1979) *The Principles of Psychiatric Rehabilitation*, Amherst, Mass., Human Resource Development Press.

ANTHONY, W. (1980) *The Skills of Diagnostic Planning*, Baltimore, Md., University Press.

ANTHONY, W. and FARKAS, M. (1982) 'A client outcome planning model for assessing psychiatric rehabilitation interventions', *Schizophrenia Bulletin*, 8, 13–38.

ANTHONY, W. and LIBERMAN, R.P. (1986) 'The practice of psychiatric rehabilitation: Historical, conceptual and research base', *Schizophrenia Bulletin*, 8, 13–38.

ANTHONY, W., COHEN, M. and VITALO, R. (1978) 'The measurement of rehabilitation outcome', *Schizophrenia Bulletin*, 4, 365–85.

BACHRACH, L.L. (1982) 'Assessment of outcome in community support systems: Results, problems and limitations', *Schizophrenia Bulletin*, 8, 39–61.

BARRIS, R., KIELHOFNER, G. and HAWKINS-WATTS, J. (1983) *Psychosocial Occupational Therapy: Practice on a Pluralistic Arena*, Laural, Md., Ramsco Publishing.

BING, R.B. (1981) 'Occupational therapy revisited: A paraphrastic journey', *American Journal of Occupational Therapy*, 35, 499–517.

BROWN, M. (1982) 'Maintenance and generalization issues in skill training with chronic schizophrenics', in CORRAN, J.P. and MONTI, P.M. (Eds), *Social Skills Training*, New York, Guildford Press, pp. 90–116.

FINE, S.B. (1980) 'Psychiatric treatment and rehabilitation: What's in a name?', *Occupational Therapy in Mental Health,* 1, 45–55.

KANTER, J.S. (1985) 'The process of change in the chronically mentally ill: A naturalistic perspective', *New Directions in Mental Health Services,* 27, 33–46.

KEATS, C.J. and MCGLASHEN, T.H. (1985) 'Intensive psychotherapy for schizophrenia', *The Yale Journal of Biology and Medicine,* 58, 239–54.

KRUPA, T. and THORNTON, J. (1986) 'The pleasure deficit in schizophrenia', *Occupational Therapy in Mental Health,* 6, 65–78.

LAMB, R.L. (1981) 'What did we really expect from deinstitutionalization?' *Hospital and Community Psychiatry,* 32, 105–9.

LAMB, R.L. (1982) *Treating the Long-Term Mentally Ill,* San Francisco, Calif., Jossey-Bass.

LIBERMAN, R.P. (1982) 'Assessment of social skills', *Schizophrenia Bulletin,* 8, 62–84.

LIBERMAN, R.P., NEUCHTERLAIN, K.H. and WALLACE, C.J. (1982) 'Social skills training and the nature of schizophrenia', in CORRAN, J.P. and MONTI, P.M. (Eds), *Social Skills Training,* New York, Guildford Press.

LIBERMAN, R.P., MASSEL, H.K., MOSK, N.D. and WON, S.E. (1985) 'Social skills training for chronic mental patients', *Hospital and Community Psychiatry,* 36, 396–403.

MALM, V. MAY, P.R. and DENCKER, S.J. (1981). 'Evaluation of the quality of life of the schizophrenia outpatient: A checklist', *Schizophrenia Bulletin,* 7, 477–87.

STERN, R. and MINKOFF, K. (1979) 'Paradoxes in programming for chronic patients in a community clinic', *Hospital and Community Psychiatry,* 30, 613–7.

STRAUSS, J.S. (1986) 'Discussion: What does rehabilitation accomplish?, *Schizophrenia Bulletin,* 12, 720–3.

WALLACE, C.J., NELSON, C.J., LIBERMAN, R.P., AITCHENSON, R.H., LUKOFF, D., ELDER, J.P. and FERSIC, C. (1980) 'A review and critique of social skills training with schizophrenic patients', *Schizophrenia Bulletin,* 6, 42–63.

Chapter 3

Occupational Therapy in General Hospital Psychiatric Units

Judith Trevan-Hawke

Although considered a 'modern' concept, psychiatric units attached to general hospitals have been in existence since the turn of the century (Prosen and Toews, 1982). There have been two major trends for developing psychiatric units attached to general hospitals:

1 a purpose-built or converted building for up to 100 beds in the grounds of or close to the parent hospital;
2 smaller units within the major hospital complex of thirty beds or less which were purpose-built or had been remodelled and refurbished during a redevelopment phase and now also with a commitment to liaison psychiatry.

The OT working in either of these settings will find the roles different from those of the OT working within the department of a large psychiatric institution. In the latter setting there are large numbers of staff from many disciplines who function from a knowledge base of psychiatry and within a multidisciplinary team approach to treatment. In the general hospital situation, however, the consulting staff, charge nurses and OTs may be the only stable personnel with a knowledge of psychiatric disorders. Therefore, patient treatment cannot become fully effective until all personnel involved with the patient have a good understanding of the philosophical approach and rationale being used by the therapist to provide treatment, thus necessitating a considerable staff education component on a regular basis to the unit in which the therapist is employed. Occupational therapists are trained to be concerned with the patient's ability to function and conform to the cultural norms of the society in which they are living with as little discomfort as possible. This entails teaching the patient to adapt or learn new skills whether the area of deficit is behavioural, emotional, cognitive or motor.

Larger psychiatric units have many similarities to the admission area of a large psychiatric hospital where there may be several OT staff who can support each other and develop programmes for greater numbers of patients from a variety of admission wards. The therapist in either setting is involved in direct patient care about 50 per cent of the working time (Connine and Hopper, 1978; Florian *et al.*, 1985). The remaining time may be spent in consultation with other disciplines, administration in relation to the case load, research to validate treatment methods and education of self, other staff and various student groups. Mosey (1981) states: 'The therapist as a consultant is not responsible for solving the presented problem — that is the responsibility of the person or group who has sought consultation' (p. 13). This is appropriate advice for the OT working in liaison psychiatry based in a general hospital where consultation to other staff and patients may be a prime aspect of the role and function.

This chapter will concentrate on the role of the OT in smaller units with a liaison component; that is, consultation to general medical patients following a psychiatrist's referral to the OT for patients with a psychological or psychosomatic overlay to their medical problem. Most of what is described can readily be transferred to those therapists working in larger but separate units from the general hospital.

The Role of Inpatient General Hospital Psychiatric Units

Individual patient treatment goals must be realistic and modest if they are to be achieved within the short period of hospitalization. Richman (1978) states, 'Patients in general hospital psychiatric units have a median stay of 12 days; 74 per cent of patients are readmissions; and many staff are involved in direct patient care' (p. 38). As patients within this setting have such a short inpatient stay, it is essential that the multidisciplinary team plans for discharge and community follow-up from admission. 'If only the care of a single [medical] practitioner were needed, hospitalisation would not be necessary' (p. 38). The mix of disciplinary expertise is essential in this short acute phase to assess and evaluate the patient's clinical state and plan for appropriate treatment which may be continued after discharge in outpatient appointments, day therapy or community support follow-up programmes.

Inpatient admission provides the opportunity to make continuous behavioural observations (Roy-Byrne *et al.*, 1986) over the twenty-four hour period by the multidisciplinary team in order to evaluate the effects of various prescribed treatment modalities. Because of the therapeutic mix of various disciplines, patients are assessed using varying perspectives rather than single professionally biased frames of reference — a situation in which the eclectically trained OT is already familiar and comfortable.

OTs, because of broadly-based training in core biopsychosocial subjects, may have to proceed cautiously in explaining their role and expertise so as not to threaten other disciplines who may feel that their work is being encroached upon. This provides an ideal opportunity for staff education regarding the philosophical approach, frame of reference and knowledge base of OT from which practice is derived. The time spent in educating staff about OT will increase the number of appropriate referrals; in many instances therapists do not see some patients because the treating team is not fully aware of the functional skills of the OT.

The concept of normality which is fostered by psychiatric patients who are admitted to general hospitals is often dispelled because, unlike large psychiatric hospitals built in rural settings with sporting facilities and park-like grounds where patients can roam at will to experience the environment, the general hospital unit will place restrictions on the residents. Patients voluntarily attending the unit may not be allowed to wander to the hospital canteen or post office without a staff escort for fear that they may intrude on the general medical care of patients in other wards and thereby disturb the fragile acceptance of psychiatric patients by some hospital personnel. This restriction of freedom may confirm a patient's fears that they are 'crazy' or 'incapable'.

The most frequently used treatments in psychiatric units are medication, physical treatments such as ECT, OT and individual or group psychotherapies using a number of approaches depending on the expertise and preference of the therapist (behavioural, analytical, person-centred, reality therapy, etc.; Corsini, 1984).

The Role of the Occupational Therapist

All the core skills learned in basic subjects such as anatomy, physiology, sociology, psychology and the advanced applied knowledge gained in studying medicine, surgery and psychiatry become the cornerstone of a holistic approach to the patient. Working within a small group of patients with psychiatric diagnoses and providing advice and education to other staff (including OTs) or patients and their families requires specialized skills in time management, observation, communication and flexibility in the choice of assessment and OT treatment regimes. The OT can be described as 'one of the few health professionals with a broad enough perspective to achieve a measure of integration of diverse data relevant to comprehensive evaluation and management of patients' (Lipowski, 1974, p. 626). All patients referred to the OT based in the psychiatric unit of a general hospital, whether a psychiatric inpatient or a patient on a general ward with a psychiatric overlay, have the same general OT principles applied to their assessment, treatment and evaluation. This highlights the importance of the therapist ensuring both medical and psychiatric registrars are fully aware of the OT contribution to the total care and well-being of the patient.

Occupational therapists are concerned with the individual's ability to perform competently in the various roles that the patient's lifestyle demands; e.g., husband/wife, father/mother, worker/recreationist in all aspects of human occupation. The therapist gathers and applies information from several levels of abstraction in relation to home, work and leisure, processes the patient's role expectations and assesses that person's ability to perform the components necessary to function at a sufficient level of expertise, thereby enabling the patient to return home whilst continuing to develop those skills in the home environment.

The role of the OT can be broken down into six components:

1 as an assessor of functional/dysfunctional performance in the patient;
2 prescribing immediate short-term treatment for easily achievable goals;
3 prescribing longer-term treatment to be carried out (a) in the admission unit, (b) by the therapist at an outpatient clinic, and (c) by referring the patient for treatment to another community-based centre which will provide more appropriate facilities.
4 as a resource person for treatment, education and social facilities available in the community for the patient and, if necessary, their family;
5 as a group leader or counsellor to inpatients, outpatients, their families and staff groups;
6 as an educator on the role and function of OT to the patient, family, staff associated with the psychiatric unit and liaison services.

On admission patients will be confused and unsure of the routine attached to the unit so time must be spent helping them to settle in and orient themselves to the venue and facilities. Once rapport between the patient and staff has begun to be established the initial OT assessment procedure either as a formal or informal interview can begin. The formal office space and usual facilities for assessment and treatment such as kitchen, quiet room and work area may have to be shared with patients and staff from the main hospital, necessitating that the psychiatric patient's social functional ability is appropriate to visiting other areas in the hospital without disrupting non-psychiatric patients' treatment programmes or causing distress to other personnel. Therefore, initial informal interviews are usually carried out on the unit or ward prior to more formalized assessments when the patient is able to leave the ward area with staff supervision. It is important that a continuum of function and dysfunction is assessed for pre-admission symptoms and behaviour as well as present functional ability. The patient's case notes or consultation with a relative or significant other will reveal pre-admission performance if the patient is unable to provide this information.

The interview is a planned conversation to elicit specific information without expecting the patient to repeat basic demographic data that can be found in the case notes. It is advisable to let patients know what prior information one has gained (e.g., age, marital status, residence) so that the subsequent questions make sense to the patient. Interview procedures (Hopkins and Smith, 1983; Shaw, 1982) whether formal or informal, enable the therapist and patient to develop treatment objectives, plan goals and establish rapport. It is important to be aware of the environment in which the interview is taking place and the degree of privacy and confidentiality that can be preserved in the inpatient ward setting. The therapist, unless she is exceptional, will probably need to take occasional notes; these should be available to the patient if requested.

The beginning therapist will need to develop interviewing skills and be able to interpret the patient's verbal and non-verbal communications in addition to being able to tolerate silences. It is important that the therapist be an active listener, able to reflect the patient's statements for verification, continually having regard for the patient's culture, age and sex norms. Biographical, past medical and family history can usually be obtained from the case notes and should not be repeated unless clarification is required. It is important at the initial interview to establish the patient's current problems, their assessment of their general health, their current living conditions and their functional ability in activities of daily living. School and occupational history as well as play and leisure inventories can be included in the initial assessment if time and fatigue level allows. However, this information can be obtained at a later time if necessary. The OT will assess the patient's ability to function using the parameters of age, competence components, time and cultural environment. Dysfunction occurring in several role behaviours and skills may not always occur on the same parameter and may therefore require differing frames of reference in the treatment process. The therapist interprets the data collated and then acts upon this information for the intervention process and treatment plan.

It is essential that clear communication occurs with patients, their families and those taking care of them whilst in the inpatient setting in order that all concerned understand the goals and priorities that patients and therapists have set. Clear communication by the therapist to individual patients as to the role of OT is an art in itself and because of the nebulous and non-assertive descriptions often given to treatment techniques and facilities, patients remain unsure of the effectiveness of OT procedures (Burton, 1984; Madden, 1984). If she is to be respected and valued for her contribution to patient management, the therapist must communicate clearly her role and treatment goals, display a sound clinical judment in the decision-making process, offer useful advice using validated assessments to support her treatment choices, and then record procedures in a comprehensible and clear manner in the case notes.

Once the initial interview and introduction to OT has been successfully completed, the therapist will be developing short-term easily achievable goals for the patient. The implementation of a treatment plan in this setting will run concurrently with further assessments and re-evaluation of the total process. A useful checklist for assessing the problem areas of patients is the Community Supports and Skills Checklist (Erickson, 1984) which, in conjunction with initial interview, will quickly highlight areas where the patient is experiencing difficulty, and therefore skills training can be implemented and evaluated during the short admission period. The checklist is made up of fifty-seven questions relating to four functional areas: physical, emotional, intellectual and interpersonal. The patient responds to the questions by indicating whether it is an asset or deficit area for them. Examples include: 'My sleeping is OK' (physical), 'I can control my anxiety' (emotional), 'I can think clearly and concentrate' (intellectual), and 'I have job interview skills' (interpersonal).

Other important inventories include: (a) The General Health Questionnaire (Creeser *et al.*, 1986); (b) Activity Configuration (Watanabe, 1968); (c) Interest Checklist (Matsutsuya, 1969); (d) Occupational Role History (Florey and Michelman, 1982); (e) Shoemyen Battery (see Hemphill, 1982); (g) Person Symbol as an Assessment Tool (King, see Hemphill, 1982); (h) Bay Area Functional Performance Evaluation (Bloomer and Williams, 1979); (i) Comprehensive Occupational Therapy Evaluation (Ehrenberg, see Hemphill, 1982); and (j) Occupational Case Analysis Interview and Rating Scale (Cubie and Kaplan, 1982). Any of these assessments can be used to evaluate the patient's function/dysfunction in a variety of performance areas and should be selected appropriately for each patient to validate treatment recommendations to the multidisciplinary team. These assessments are also used for evaluation and discussion with the patient to establish and enhance self-understanding, to develop personal growth skills through discussion of performance levels in the assessments and to reduce or prevent maladaptive coping behaviours such as temper tantrums or violence.

The OT working with a commitment to liaison psychiatry must also be able to operate effectively by having a sound basic knowledge in the discipline and having a genuine balance of the arts and science which can then be integrated into the unique configuration which comprises OT. Elliot (1981) has expressed similar philosophical aims for psychiatrists working in the psychiatric liaison area.

The multi-diagnostic group of liaison patients that may be referred to the OT will most likely have had full psychological and psychiatric assessment by the referring psychiatrist and a specific referral for a treatment modality will be described; that is, if the therapist has previously initiated adequate education to the referring psychiatrist as to the skills and expertise of the OT. These treatment techniques are usually brief and can be conducted by the therapist in the general ward situation, the main OT department if the physical condition of the patient allows moving them, or the psychiatric ward. In these situations treatment can be done individually with the liaison patient or if applicable with a group of psychiatric inpatients. Techniques most likely to be used by the OT are behaviour modification, pain reduction, biofeedback, guided imagery, sleep management, relaxation, self-hypnosis and meditation. Specific modalities are selected for patients according to their psychiatric and medical problems and these are usually described as skills or techniques that patients can utilize for their own benefit once discharged. If necessary, patients may return as outpatients for additional reinforcement of treatment techniques. Those patients requiring longer admission for extended physical examination or treatment procedures to alleviate illnesses whose problems are mainly neurotic may use other OT treatments such as expressive art, music and technical crafts depending on time available.

The holistic approach to psychiatry in general hospitals suits the OT's eclectic background and supports the knowledge that preventative medicine can be enhanced through education and advice to a variety of patients either individually or in groups, particularly to those patients who are prepared to access OT outpatient facilities. The benefits of diet, exercise, positive mental attitude and the role of a strong belief system to support the individual through times of crisis or stress (Pasnau, 1982) are part of the OT's basic treatment approach in this varied caseload. The therapist working in psychiatry will include psychodynamic, somatic and economic factors as components of the assessment and treatment plan.

Group therapy has been shown to be useful for special groups (other than in the traditionally accepted psychiatric area) such as survivors of myocardial infarction where depression and phobic responses to work and sex are reduced in comparisons to control subjects not attending support groups (Rahe, 1979). Depression is the commonest psychiatric disorder encountered in liaison patient referrals. Other deviant behaviours may include self-destructive non-compliance with medical advice, excessive dependence on the hospital or personnel, gross denial of the illness, a 'given-up' attitude or suicide attempts or threats (Lipowski, 1974). Liaison psychiatry adheres to the psychosomatic approach, and reasons that human health and disease result from an interaction of biological, psychological and social factors reflecting the training and rationale for treatment by the OT. Such a variety of diagnoses is rarely found in any other branch of psychiatry and creates a stimulating environment in which the therapist can develop many skills. Lipowski (1967) describes the satisfactions of working in liaison psychiatry where the therapist's total knowledge base is used: 'Prompt and dramatic gains can be seen in patients in comparison to the slower progress seen in traditional psychiatric settings' (p. 159).

Community Care Preparation and Follow-up

The OT will have assessed each patient to ensure that on discharge they will be able to cope with society and the community facilities within their cultural environment regardless of whether the patient is returning to live alone, with the family, to another hospital, or sheltered or residential accommodation. As culturally/environmentally appropriate, each patient participates in activities which allow them to demonstrate their competence in using public or private transport, shopping/budgetting and self-care skills, the use of banks, post office, public houses/bars, cinema, church, cafes and evening classes (Wykes *et al.*, 1982). The OT programme provides training in social, leisure or work skills, or elements of these as required. Some patients will be transferred to larger psychiatric inpatient facilities while others are referred to day hospital or community support services for continuing care, treatment and assessment.

The close proximity of general hospitals to towns and cities with good public transport systems enables community assessment and training programmes to be instituted more readily than in the remote parent psychiatric institution. However, in general hospital psychiatric units restrictions on leaving the hospital may be imposed because of the difficulties in organizing visiting specialists from other disciplines who arrive to assess organic or physical conditions in the psychiatric patient, the arrangement of medical tests in other departments (e.g., CAT scans), and because an outing reduces staff numbers on the ward. These frustrations can be overcome if the OT carefully organizes the practical assessment and clearly communicates the purpose and rationale for the outing to all relevant personnel. Trust and confidence in the therapist by other disciplines will depend on the therapist's skill at communicating and educating the team members on the importance and relevance of such assessments.

Waryszak (1982) conducted a follow-up study of sixty-one patients after discharge from a psychiatric unit attached to a general hospital, finding that one month after discharge there was a considerable improvement in symptomatology and social adjustment. However, at four weeks post-discharge, there was no further change in social adjustment although improvements in social and leisure activities usage had occurred. The patient's level of social adjustment did not reach the same level as the community sample group, while symptomatology had continued to decrease. This study highlights the importance of achieving optimum pre-discharge competence in these functional activities so as to maintain the patient in the community for as long as possible.

Family and social supports can be maintained and encouraged more easily in a psychiatric unit because of easy access to the hospital by transport. Patient and families may feel that there is less stigma attached to a general hospital where one need not state which ward the patient is going to. Neighbours and acquaintances who might censure psychiatric behaviour are more accepting if they believe, even erroneously, that the patient's behaviour has an organic or physical origin. Education of the public as to the true nature of psychiatric illness and the way it manifests itself in individuals is not the sole responsibility of the OT, but they can contribute significantly in this sphere. The therapist may frequently be asked to explain symptoms, behaviours and treatment procedures to families and friends of a patient as well as speaking to public groups in nationally organized health weeks, or at self-help group meetings. This is in addition to in-service sessions within the main hospital complex to interdisciplinary groups.

Occupational Therapy in Liaison Psychiatry: Problems and Solutions

Although psychiatric units in general hospitals are not a new concept, the proportion of OTs working in this area is still quite small, and even fewer are attached to a liaison psychiatry team. Because of the uncertainty of other hospital personnel as to the role and function of the staff in the psychiatry unit, in particular the role of the psychiatric OT in a general hospital, there are inherent problems. These problems are compounded by the changes in policy of national and state institutions to restrict admission, reduce length of stay in hospital, and increase the number of community support facilities available to long-term or chronic psychiatric patients. In reality there are high readmission rates for deinstitutionalized patients, often to a pyschiatric unit attached to a general hospital. These units were originally built to provide evaluation and crisis treatment for the acutely ill but now find that a proportion of the admitted patients are homeless and chronically ill (Schoonover and Bassuk, 1983).

The difficulties of non-psychiatrically trained staff and frequent rotations have already been mentioned but can be alleviated to some extent by education. For permanent staff based in the unit the revolving door syndrome of patient admissions may lead to confusion over their expected and actual care-giving role. They 'cannot refuse care of admission to the generally lower socioeconomic, unwanted segment of the psychiatric population' (Blotnick-Pender, 1984, p. 132). This can lead to an inadequate amount of the time being spent with the patient and an increase in the number of decision-making meetings to cope with personal frustration and low morale. When staff conflict and confusion arise in psychiatric units of a general hospital, where there are small numbers or only one member of a profession working within the team, the group's defence may be to deny the internal aggression and direct these feelings onto an identified enemy. This can be a patient, a relative or a visiting staff member. 'Burnout' is often the explanation given for the despair and lack of ego integrity displayed and should be challenged and ameliorated quickly. The psychiatric inpatient service is usually managed on the same lines as non-psychiatric services despite vastly differing needs. The leadership follows the autocratic medical model and when the leader is absent for lengthy periods the group may become disorganized and relatively unstructured, reducing the functioning capacity of the group and increasing the levels of emotionality. The OT's knowledge of psychology and sociology can assist comprehension of group dynamics and provide an opportunity to help other members in the staff group to recognize the signs of disintegration and reduced functioning for patient treatment.

If the treatment team is to remain a cohesive group it is important to have organized in-service education programmes and staff support groups. Despite staff turnover, individuals on the team can be assisted to feel secure and stable in this environment. When difficult patients have complex problems or management disorders become an issue on the unit, the opportunity to discuss and debrief as a staff group enhances group problem-solving and disseminates the information as well as educating less experienced staff. Regular in-service programmes should be instituted not only to ensure that all team members are aware of the role of their colleagues but also to introduce new as well as familiar techniques and treatment approaches for patient care. These sessions not only enable staff to develop new skills and increase their knowledge base but also offer an opportunity to discuss real or imagined clinical inadequacies in themselves. As a cohesive team, the staff can more adequately cope with the frustrations incurred because of the lack of community follow-up facilities and lobby the hospital management to make provisions where there is a recognized shortfall in patient services. Schoonover and Bassuk (1983) state that a similar programme in the USA increased the team's involvement in patient aftercare. Outpatient therapists, family, friends and community resources were involved earlier and more vigorously in the treatment and increased the staff's ability to treat a wider range of patients. Staff became more contented and were able to institute a rehabilitation approach for those patients requiring longer-term contact with the hospital.

In spite of the difficulties of working as an OT in this environment, there are many rewards in terms of working with several different diagnoses, and treating both physical and psychiatric disorders in patients. The ability to develop good interdisciplinary communication skills and education programmes for a wide variety of areas is essential. Bachrach (1981) has stated that 'general hospital psychiatry shows astonishingly great vitality. There is ample evidence that the field continues to initiate and evaluate varied and imaginative treatment strategies, to develop and improve programmes of brief hospitalization for crisis intervention, to develop innovative training procedures and unusual collaborative service arrangements, and to engage in productive research' (p. 880).

The Future

Because of their biosocial training, OTs are ideally suited to work as team members on a psychiatric unit of a general hospital and should be developing and expanding this field. The prime area for OT expansion is in prevention; by providing day or outpatient support services through individual or group counselling and specific skill groups such as relaxation, social skills and assertiveness training. With the increase in unemployment and early retirement the OT is the skilled member of the team who can develop programmes to increase skills in leisure planning and stress reduction programmes. There are many personal and professional gains from working within such a setting. Many hospitals now offer OT outpatient services to enhance continuity of care and follow-up by a key therapist. Some psychiatric emergency services encourage the OT (when known to the service and rostered in this way) to contribute to the patient's assessment at a walk-in clinic or telephone crisis service, suicide prevention centre or a home visit programme. These are more unusual examples of how the OT's skills may be developed to cope with expanding services, but they are areas into which OTs with specialized skills have embarked and developed programmes, thereby gaining respect for their expertise and professionalism.

References

BACHRACH, L.L. (1981) 'General hospital psychiatry: Overview from a sociological perspective', *American Journal of Psychiatry,* 138, 879–87.

BLOOMER, J. and WILLIAMS, S. (1979) *The Bay Area Functional Performance Evaluation,* San Francisco, Calif., Langley Porter Institute.

BLOTNICK-PENDER, V.S. (1984) 'Institutional pathology in a psychiatric inpatient service', *Psychiatric Quarterly,* 56, 130–7.

BURTON, L. (1984) 'Introducing the concept of occupational therapy to patients in an acute psychiatric unit', *British Journal of Occupational Therapy,* 47, 178–83.

CONNINE, T.A. and HOPPER, D.L. (1978) 'Work sampling: A tool in management', *American Journal of Occupational Therapy,* 32, 301–4.

CORSINI, R.J. (1984) *Current Psychotherapies,* 3rd ed., New York Peacock Books.

CREESER, R.A., GOOCH, A. and WIGGINS, R.D. (1986) 'An evaluation of the effectiveness of the general health questionnaire in an occupational therapy setting', *British Journal of Occupational Therapy,* 49, 39–41.

CUBIE, S. and KAPLAN, K. (1982) 'A case analysis method for the model of occupation', *American Journal of Occupational Therapy,* 36, 645–56.

EHRENBERG, F. (1982) 'Comprehensive assessment process: A group evaluation', in HEMPHILL, B. (Ed.), *The Evaluative Process in Psychiatric Occupational Therapy,* Thorofare, N. J., Charles B. Slack

ELLIOT, R.S. (1981) 'Environmental and behavioural influences in the major cardiovascular disorders', in WEISS, S. *et al.* (Eds), *Perspectives on Behavioural Medicine,* New York, Academic Press.

ERICKSON, R.C. (1984) 'Psychosocial assessment on a short-stay inpatient psychiatric unit', *Psychological Reports,* 55, 43–7.

FOREY, L.L. and MICHELMAN, S.M. (1982) 'Occupational role history: A screening tool for psychiatric occupational therapy', *American Journal of Occupational Therapy,* 36, 301–8.

FLORIAN, V., SHAFFER, M. and SACHS, D. (1985) 'Time allocation patterns of occupational therapists in Israel: Implications for job satisfaction', *American Journal of Occupational Therapy,* 39, 392–6.

HEMPHILL, B.J. (1982) *The Evaluation Process in Psychiatric Occupational Therapy,* Thorofare, N.J., Charles B. Slack.

HOPKINS, H.L.L. and SMITH, H.D. (1983) *Willard and Spackman's Occupational Therapy,* 6th ed., Philadelphia, Pa., J.B. Lippincott.

LERNER, C. (1982) 'The magazine picture collage', in HEMPHILL, B. (Ed.), *The Evaluative Process in Psychiatric Occupational Therapy,* Thorofarc, N.J., Charles B. Slack.

LIPOWSKI, Z.J. (1967) 'Review of consultation psychiatry and psychosomatic medicine', *Psychosomatic Medicine,* 29, 153–71.

LIPOWSKI, Z.J. (1974) 'Consultation-liaison psychiatry: An overview', *American Journal of Psychiatry,* 131, 623–30.

MADDEN, A. (1984) 'Explaining psychiatric occupational therapy: An art in itself: *British Journal of Occupational Therapy,* 47, 15–7.

MATSUTSUYA, J.S. (1969) 'The interest checklist', *American Journal of Occupational Therapy,* 23, 323–8.

MOSEY, A.C. (1981) *Occupational Therapy: Configuration of a Profession,* New York, Raven Press.

PASNAU, R.O. (1982) 'Consultation-liaison psychiatry at the crossroads: In search of a definition for the 1980s', *Hospital and Community Psychiatry,* 33, 989–95.

PROSEN, H. and TOEWS, J. (1982) 'Psychiatric units under analysis', *Dimensions in Mental Health*, 4, 30–3.

RAHE, R.H., WARD, H.W. and HAYES, V. (1979) 'Brief group therapy in myocardial infarction rehabilitation: Three-to-four-year follow-up of a controlled trial', *Psychosomatic Medicine,* 41, 229–42.

RICHMAN, A. (1978) 'Quality assurance, PSRO and the medical record for psychiatric patients', *Medical Record News,* 49, 38–41.

ROY-BYRNE, P., PYNOOS, R.S. and GLICK, I.D. (1986) 'The inpatient psychiatric unit as consultation service', *Canadian Journal of Psychiatry,* 31, 54–8.

SCHOONOVER, S.C. and BASSUK, E.L. (1983) 'Deinstitutionalization and the private general hospital inpatient unit: Implications for clinical care', *Hospital and Community Psychiatry,* 34, 135–9.

SHAW, C. (1982) 'The interview process', in HEMPHILL, B.J. (Ed.), *The Evaluative Process in Psychiatric Occupational Therapy,* Thorofare, N.J., Charles B. Slack.

SHOEMYEN, C.W. (1982) The Shoemyen battery, in HEMPHILL, B.J. (Ed.), *The Evaluative Process in Psychiatric Occupational Therapy,* Thorofare, N.J., Charles B. Slack.

WARYSZAK, Z. (1982) 'Symptomatology and social adjustment of psychiatric patients before and after hospitalisation', *Social Psychiatry,* 17, 149–54.

WATANABE, S. (1968) 'Activities configuration', *1968 Regional Institute on the Evaluation Process: Final Report,* RSA 123T68, New York, American Occupational Therapy Association.

WYKES, Y., STURT, E. and CREER, C. (1982) 'Practices of day and residential units in relation to the social behaviour of attenders', in WING, J.K. (Ed.), *Psychological Medicine,* Monograph Supplement 2, 15–27.

Chapter 4

Occupational Therapy in Psychiatric Day-Treatment

Kathleen Griffith Hoehn

The concept of the acute psychiatric day-treatment is a comparatively new addition to the mental health care system. Day-treatment is a voluntary, short-term, multidisciplinary programme providing an alternative approach to adults with emotional disturbances. A psychiatric partial hospitalization (day-treatment) is frequently recommended to individuals who require a level of care that exceeds outpatient services in frequency and degree of structure. However, day-treatment is less intense, protective and restrictive than most inpatient psychiatric settings. For many, day-treatment is a transitional form of treatment which follows inpatient hospitalization to further progress and provide support for the return to community and private living situations.

The programme encourages independence, personal responsibility and self-esteem, while providing a structured environment, emotional support and stimulation for positive change. A psychodynamic emphasis and multidisciplinary approach can provide stabilization for acute situations and improvement of coping skills for those with longer-term problems.

Occupational Therapist Role

The OT's areas of specialization include evaluation and assessment of the patient in the OT setting, establishment of a therapeutic relationship, treatment planning and the development of an OT treatment programme. The OT, using the information gathered in the evaluation and assessment, is responsible for directing and structuring individual group activity sessions and working towards the designated therapeutic goals.

Fidler and Fidler (1978) state that the word 'doing' is selected to convey the sense of performing, producing or causing. Doing is the process of investigating, trying out, and gaining evidence of one's capacity for experiencing, responding, managing, creating and controlling. It is through such feedback from both the non-human and human objects that an individual comes to know the potential and limitations of self and the environment and achieves a sense of competence and instrinsic worth. The primary objective of an activity session is to direct action-oriented activities and to provide a therapeutic arena for the actual doing of a particular task. Focusing on the 'here and now' and reality aspects of the situation provides an opportunity to work towards goals as opposed to verbalizing goals and to identify the problems which interfere with the completion of a task. Following the activity session, the OT and the patient can discuss experiences sustained during the work and apply these to an examination of individual treatment goals. Generally, patients gain a better understanding of their interests, needs, capacities and limitations. As a result of engaging in new activities, patients gain awareness of the correspondence to parallel life situations and develop insight and improved coping skills.

So often we hear the phrase 'actions speak louder than words'. OT activity sessions provide the environment and experiences in the day-treatment setting where this maxim can be explored, discussed and evaluated. A patient's functioning level in the programme is generally an accurate reflection of their personality style and functioning ability outside the programme. The OT uses observations made in the session to assist patients in identifying the similarities between their experiences working within the activities setting and their difficulties outside the programme. It is through this interaction that patients learn to recognize their own patterns of thinking, feeling and relating. Their actions, demonstrated in the session, accurately portray both the hopes for change and growth and the discrepancies of fear and resistance.

Individual Occupational Therapy Sessions

Upon admission to the programme the patient is asked to complete an initial OT orientation procedure. The initial orientation consists of a magazine picture collage, perceptual screening test and identification of treatment goals. During the orientation and interview which follows, the therapist establishes a supportive therapeutic rapport, gathers information necessary for evaluation and clarifies initial treatment goals. All of this information will be useful in designing a treatment approach which will best meet the patient's needs, interests and abilities.

Fidler (1981) states in 'From crafts to competence' that to put the fundamental concepts of OT into practice, we must have a broad repertoire of activity 'know how'. We must have the expertise to know the why, the what, the when and the how of activities. Also the importance of matching a given activity with an individual's readiness to learn, ability to receive stimuli, values, norms and personal characteristics at a real and symbolic level will determine the quality of satisfaction, motivation, development, learning and remediation.

Therapeutic Relationship

Requisite to all forms of treatment and therapy is the establishment of a supportive therapeutic relationship between the individual and the therapist. This positive, supportive relationship is characterized by trust, concern, acceptance, empathy, understanding and open communication. Acceptance of the patient as an individual without a hidden agenda to change him/her is a principle which the OT needs to be conscientiously aware of at all times. A desire to change someone precludes acceptance, and change poses a threat to many, especially to the patient who has developed a fragile way of relating. The threatened individual will respond with resistance and this will present many barriers in the therapeutic process. If patients feel accepted as they are, they gain the freedom to stay that way or make a new choice. Through supportive confrontation and acceptance, patients' survival and defence mechanisms may be exposed but they are not criticised or ripped away leaving them defenceless. If these mechanisms cause too much pain, they can decide on their own volition to give up but first they have to be aware and experience them clearly. Acceptance helps patients see themselves clearly and make that decision (Dunning, 1973).

Activity and Craft Selection

Upon completion of the initial orientation, interview, clarification of treatment goals and establishment of the therapeutic rapport, the patient actively chooses a project to initiate. Ongoing evaluation of the patient's task skills will be made during work on the initial project. Independent decision-making is encouraged throughout, although the therapist will make recommendations on a discriminate basis. Using previously obtained information, the therapist will present input regarding the choice of project if it is contrary to the patient's initial treatment goals and functioning level.

Due to the critically important initial stage of the therapeutic relationship, early project recommendations and directions are minimal. Activities are not mandated so the patient is faced with the necessity to choose what he will or will not do. The environment is shaped but the patient must define himself, his preferences, and his skills by personal choice (Dunning, 1973).

Crafts as the Catalytic Agent

Using craft activities as a catalytic agent in an acute day-treatment setting is a highly useful, dynamic and therapeutic mode of treatment. The use of craft activities and exploration of the 'here and now' situations provide a tremendous opportunity to gain awareness, insight and understanding into successful experiences which increase self-esteem and reveal problem areas which inhibit or present barriers towards obtaining therapeutic goals.

The following sections will define and describe how the patient selects OT goals and problem areas. Table 4.1 can be utilized when using crafts or activities as the therapeutic agent. Therapeutic recommendations, ideas and approaches are addressed. Using their knowledge of human behaviour and psychiatric understanding, the therapist can adjust her approach accordingly and parallel the problem areas experienced during the session. The therapeutic objective is to foster understanding, insight and coping in specific problem areas and emotional difficulties.

For the enhancement of self-understanding to occur the therapist needs to explore and establish a treatment plan with the individual as to how their personal goals can be addressed during the session. During the initial interview and ongoing interaction, the therapist and patient can explore and discuss patterns of behaviour exhibited while working on projects as related to goals and other identified therapeutic issues.

Self-Esteem and Confidence

Self-esteem is a state of being on good terms with one's self. In more classical terms having good self-esteem is functioning without the fear of self-criticism, punishment or abandonment. Self-confidence is a belief in one's own abilities and competencies. When motivation, ability or self-confidence is decreased, participation in any activity feels very risky. Most patients approach the doing of activities therapy with tremendous fears about their own competency and a limited belief in their ability to control their environment. The essential features of patients exhibiting low self-esteem and decreased self-confidence in an OT session are an inability to recognize or measure accomplishments, self-deprecating or derogatory comments, magnification of errors, inability to receive compliments, decreased

Table 4.1. Occupational Therapy Goals and Problem Areas.

Occupational therapy is a therapeutic programme designed for you during your involvement at Day Hospital. Our primary goal is to assist you in developing or increasing your skills to help you feel more positive about yourself and to enjoy a more productive life. As an individual, your treatment programme may differ from others according to your needs. You and your occupational therapist will be working together to select tasks designed to help you accomplish your goals.

Please check three or four of the following which most apply to you.

( ) I would like to improve my self-esteem and confidence.
( ) I want to be more comfortable with people and improve my ability to relate to others.
( ) I want to be more assertive and communicate in a positive way.
( ) I want to be able to set goals, and follow through decisions.
( ) I would like to be able to structure my time more effectively so that I can accomplish my goals.
( ) I want to have more energy and motivation.
( ) I want to be more independent.
( ) I would like to be able to problem-solve more effectively.
( ) I would like to develop new interests and explore my use and abuse of leisure time.
( ) I would like to be able to identify my feelings and improve my ability to cope and channel my emotions more constructively.
( ) I need to learn to think things through before I act impulsively.
( ) I want to learn when it is appropriate to seek assistance.
( ) I want to be more organized, and improve my attention and concentration.
( ) I would like to ....

Source: Sinai Hospital, Detroit.

risk-taking behaviour, resistance to making projects for one's self, and the seeking of approval from others. When an individual has low self-esteem, they are often very involved in a dependent style of interaction and rely on outside approval. As a result, they will frequently seek out suggestions, opinions and ideas about their own decisions. These patients' needs for reassurance and guidance are unrelenting.

The fundamental issue in all initial contacts with the patient is the establishment of a therapeutic relationship and acceptance and understanding of the person's issues of concern. After a basic level of trust has been established, the therapist may begin to confront the individual about observed patterns of behaviour. These problems touch on sensitive feelings and the exploration of observed patterns of behaviour may cause defensiveness or resistance. The therapist needs to understand these feelings and be ready to adjust the approach supportively in order to maintain a positive interaction.

A significant therapeutic area for dealing with problems of self-esteem centres on the dependent individual's characteristic pattern of making decisions. The therapist needs to encourage the individual to make decisions based on their needs, feelings and desires. Although dependent persons will seek constant assistance to make their decisions, it is important for the therapist to redirect and reinforce independent decision-making. Assisting others to make decisions may result in facilitating the dependency and increasing the person's feelings of incompetence.

Interpersonal Skills and Relationships with Others

The quality of an individual's interpersonal skills is determined by their degree of comfort with people and ability to trust others. Past and present relationships form the basis for the nature and style of the individual's future relationships, and influence beliefs and attitudes about one's self and others. When a person feels uncomfortable or ill-at-ease around others, their ability to relate openly and spontaneously will be inhibited. Any kind of social situation or interaction which increases this internal discomfort will increase anxiety and decrease the person's sense of internal stability. These individuals are likely to feel very vulnerable and experience fears of rejection, loss of personal power and control, and feelings of inadequacy. Very often, due to the anxiety and feelings of vulnerability, problems with communication accompany difficulties with interpersonal relationships.

Common observations and associated behaviours of this problem manifested in the OT setting include isolation, withdrawal, avoidance, decreased spontaneous interaction, superficial and guarded self-disclosure, minimal verbalization and increased anxiety when approached by others. There is a great variance in the pattern of anxiety responses seen in individuals. For example, changes may be observed in the areas of flow of speech, facial expression, eye contact, expressive movements of the hands and postural changes.

When communication styles are antagonistic to the development of personal relationships, the therapeutic approach needs to reinforce appropriate limits and boundaries. Persons need to become respectful to individuals and materials. Role modelling and supportive confrontations are useful ways of demonstrating and placing limits on styles of relating which facilitate interpersonal relationships. Topics of discussion need to reflect awareness of the communication style, reactions and feelings evoked in others, and the long-range implication of maintaining this style of relating.

When individuals are inhibited in their capacity to relate openly, supportive therapeutic methods can be initiated to facilitate interpersonal interactions. These methods may include questioning, initiating discussion of topics to stimulate verbalization of the group as a whole, seating arrangements which decrease the opportunity for isolation and withdrawal, and group activities. Utilization of group activities may stimulate and facilitate social interactions based on common interests and experiences.

Increasing Assertiveness and Positive Communication

Communication is the process of conveying ideas, emotions, attitudes and actions from one person to another. The four basic styles of communication are assertive, passive, aggressive, and passive-aggressive.

Assertive communication. This is a style which involves direct expression of thoughts, feelings and actions in a manner which is respectful to both the communicator's rights and the rights of others. It facilitates meaningful relationships and promotes further communication and positive feelings. Assertive communication can be characterized by a non-confiding ability to express feelings, exchange information, seek assistance and compromise on areas of disagreement.

Passive communication. This is the failure to communicate one's feelings, needs and desires, and it is frequently disrespectful to the communicator's rights. Individuals who communicate in a passive style have difficulty recognizing and expressing their feelings and needs. Consequently other people tend to respond with a similar lack of consideration for the passive person resulting from their experience of frustration and unresponsiveness. An example might be a common response of passive indifference when asked for their opinions or feelings. This pattern of unresponsiveness will result in others decreasing their consideration of the passive individual.

Aggressive communication. This form is an expression of feelings, thoughts and desires in a manner which remain disrespectful to the rights of others and also to the communicator himself. It can be characterized by harsh verbal language, inconsiderate and provocative interactions with others, accusations of others or name calling. Aggressive body language can include throwing objects, slamming doors, pointing of the index finger, abrupt body movements, clenched teeth and glaring of the eyes.

Passive-aggressive communication. This involves the expression of feelings, primarily anger, in a manner which is indirect and disrespectful to the rights of others. Behaviours and personality characteristics associated with passive-aggressive communication include sarcasm, attention-seeking behaviours, belittling the activity and procrastinating. These individuals have a tendency to use non-verbal language and attention-seeking behaviours in an astute manner. Instead of verbalizing their need for assistance, they may draw attention through audible means by letting out a deep sigh, abruptly leaving the area or roughly pushing their project away. Upon approach or when offering assistance after an episode of non-verbal acting out, it is important to clarify verbally the meaning behind the indirect message.

The initial therapeutic objective is to discuss and identify the problem areas as they relate to the individual's communication style and identified treatment goal. Exploration of the barriers to assertive communication can be helpful to clarify further the specific underlying areas of difficulty. Some of the obstacles to direct communication may be a fear of rejection, low self-esteem and issues of control.

When dealing with passive communication styles, the objective is to offer support, and to encourage and provide the opportunity for expression of feelings and assertive communication to occur. Recommended therapeutic techniques are for the therapist supportively to structure their approach and the environment to encourage interaction with others, verbalization and seeking of assistance.

When dealing with aggressive communication styles, it is helpful to explore the situations and feelings which precipitated the aggressive communication. The individual and therapist need to identify constructive alternatives of coping with similar or anticipated situations which may occur in the setting. Supportively, the individual and the therapist are both setting appropriate limits for respectful and constructive communication to occur.

Many individuals in the day-treatment programme identify with the goal of wanting to be more assertive and to communicate in a positive way. Although individuals frequently are able to identify their specific communication style, they lack the necessary awareness and insight to take risks and venture outside their repetitive pattern of relating. The therapeutic focus is to assist with increasing one's awareness and explore the underlying areas of difficulty which present barriers and serve to maintain current communication style.

Setting Goals and Following through Decisions

The ability to make decisions is comprised of the ability to choose a desired alternative regarding a specific dispute or question. Setting a goal is having an aim or objective to which actions, thoughts and feelings are directed.

Setting goals and following through decisions entail being able to identify what one is striving to obtain and persisting with effort to achieve the identified goal. Individuals who have difficulty setting goals frequently acknowledge being unable to make up their mind and they remain uncertain and perplexed when presented with problems. They are often unable to commit themselves to a specific goal. Behaviours and personality characteristics associated with difficulties in setting goals including ambivalence, vagueness, dependency, indecisiveness, resistance, perfectionism and fear of failure.

Difficulty following through with decisions is another common problem area. Individuals will report decreased perseverance to achieve goals. The actual behaviours demonstrated are not consistent with their stated goals. They will complain about decreased motivation, difficulty with initiation, losing interest and not being able to cope with problems which may arise while working towards a goal. During the OT session persons may choose not to continue their project and request initiation of a new one. Generally it is due to poor frustration tolerance or loss of interest based on initial impulsive decisions. Behaviours and personality characteristics associated with this problem area include impulsivity, poor ability to concentrate, procrastination, critical assessment of actions based on perfectionistic standards and low frustration tolerance.

Due to the nature of the OT sessions, there is a great opportunity to acknowledge this problem area. Participation in individual sessions entails selecting an activity of choice and working on the desired project until completion. The recommended therapeutic approach is to discuss the problems encountered by the individual in the activity and to draw parallels to similar life situations. When individuals have problems with making decisions, they will frequently manipulate others to make their decisions. They will seek advice and request others' input to solve problems and make their decisions. The therapeutic idea is to place limits and redirect the individual to encourage independent decision-making based on the person's needs, feelings and desires.

When dealing with problems of decreased follow-through, it is helpful to explore, discuss and increase awareness of the underlying areas of conflict. The person is encouraged to express feelings with alternative coping mechanisms explored to facilitate follow-through and increase frustration tolerance.

Structuring Time Effectively and Accomplishing Goals

Individuals who have difficulty in this problem area frequently identify decreased life functioning, a diminished sense of accomplishment and an inability to complete tasks. They will complain about frustrated ambitions and of being unable to complete the goals which they state are important. Very often they will report feeling out of control in their use of time and express a desire for more organization in their lives. These individuals often feel depressed with anger focused on themselves. They are aware of their difficulties in managing time, their actions and energy expenditures.

Common behaviours of this problem area are manifested in the OT setting and include difficulties with initiating activities, allowing adequate time to pursue goals, and inability to prioritize actions. During the activity session they arrive late, use the session unproductively, become easily distracted, lose interest and request a change in their choice of project prior to its completion. During periods of increased stress individuals frequently choose not to work on their projects and remain unstructured throughout the session. Common difficulties for these individuals can include dependency on others and outside controls to structure their time, ambivalence, undecisiveness, helplessness, feeling overwhelmed, thought preoccupation, decreased motivation, limited energy and resistance.

The therapeutic emphasis when exploring issues related to this problem area is on increasing one's awareness of the inconsistencies between stated goals and the actual behaviour demonstrated towards their achievement. What a person does to reach their goals is often different from the verbalized desire of a goal. The therapeutic idea is to explore the underlying areas of conflict and identify patterns of behaviour observed in the setting as they relate to the problem area. Frequently, the inherent structure of the setting allows for successful follow-through and accomplishment of goals. If this is the case, recommended discussion would centre on identifying ways in which the individuals could provide structure outside the setting to increase the opportunity for follow-through and accomplishment of goals.

Improving Energy and Motivation

This problem area has a tendency to touch all aspects of life. In dealing with this area the therapeutic idea is to assist the individual to become aware that increased activity can also increase energy and motivation. Individuals experiencing a lack of motivation, energy and interest present a difficult therapeutic challenge. The author's practical experience predicts that increased activity will result in increased motivation and interest, yet these individuals lack sufficient motivation for the initiation of the therapeutic activity. The recommended approach is to explore and discuss the advantages and disadvantages of decreased activity and identify the person's individual responsibility regarding the choice of their behaviour.

Participation in an activity can provide an opportunity for accomplishments of pleasurable feelings. Although there is no guarantee that pleasurable feelings will result, due to past experience there is a level of predictability that the negative feelings will persist if no action is taken to deal with them differently. It is advisable to discuss the problems encountered by the person in the activity and to draw parallels to similar life situations. Frequently there are many self-defeating patterns of behaviours associated with this problem area. Individuals will complain that tasks appear too great and no effort will bring them any closer to their goals. Encouraging the person to address one aspect at a time can be helpful as opposed to the entirety which is overwhelming, depressing and self-defeating. Procrastination is another significant area related to decreased energy and motivation. When individuals procrastinate, a tremendous amount of time and mental energy is spent in putting off doing things. Procrastination becomes self-defeating when the person's self-deprecating thoughts increase due to lack of action.

Independence

Independence is a state of being free from the influence or control of others. When individuals function independently they are comfortable with relying on their own judgments. They trust their ability to make decisions and resolve conflicts. Dependent individuals have difficulty making decisions and functioning autonomously due to their decreased capacity to assume responsibility for their lives. These individuals rely heavily on the influence, control and decision-making abilities of others.

The therapeutic objects are to encourage and support independent thinking, decision-making, problem-solving and behaviours. The consistent therapeutic approach will provide opportunities for increased awareness of the problem, personal responsibility, self-reliance and independent functioning. Dependent individuals require constant redirection, encouragement and support from the therapist to tolerate the opportunities for increasing independent behaviours. With supportive limits maintained to increase independent functioning, it is common for individuals to experience frustration and anger. These emotions increase the likelihood of acting out behaviour in the session. The person is experiencing feelings and reacting to their unmet dependency needs. The recommended therapeutic approach is to encourage verbalization of feeling and explore constructive ways of coping which are realistic to the setting.

Problem-solving

Problem-solving is being able to deal with and resolve questions which are presented for solutions. Individuals who have difficulty in this problem area frequently identify not being able to come up with solutions, feeling overwhelmed, not tolerating problem situations, and selecting solutions which do not resolve the problem. Very often they will report that their manner of problem-solving is repetitive and predictable, although it does not aid them in adapting to conflict. These individuals commonly experience a high degree of frustration because of their ineffectual ways of dealing with the problem.

How one copes with problems which arise during activities is generally an accurate reflection of how one handles and reacts to problems outside the setting. Initially the therapist needs to clarify if the difficulties with problem-solving are long-standing areas of conflict or specific to the individual's current level of functioning and emotional difficulty. For example, a depressed individual may become overwhelmed and unable to resolve problems during emotional difficulties although reports past abilities to handle similar situations with ease. Some individuals will state that although their ability to problem-solve is currently diminished, it also was an area of difficulty prior to the depression. Clarifying this concept will provide information regarding the person's problem-solving abilities and suggest realistic treatment expectations to be achieved in an acute setting. If the problem area is reflective of the person's emotional difficulty, it is reasonable to anticipate improvements in problem-solving as the emotional difficulties lessen. If the problem-solving is a long-standing area of conflict, improvements will be noted although they will be less significant due to the deeply ingrained and life-long behavioural patterns.

The therapeutic emphasis is to discuss behaviours observed, facilitate awareness of problem-solving techniques, and supportively explore options and alternatives. Presenting themselves in helpless fashion, the dependent person will require firm redirection to make decisions and to problem-solve independently. The low functioning individual, who is unable to problem-solve independently, will benefit from a more structured approach. The therapist can assist with focusing alternatives and presenting selected options. The person is then encouraged to make decisions independently based on information received.

Use and Abuse of Leisure Time

This problem area refers to what a person does and how they use their time which is free and unstructured. Many individuals report having difficulty with identifying or satisfying their personal needs. They will report feeling bored, idle, lonely, withdrawn or agitated during periods of decreased structure or unoccupied time. Leisure interests which remain unfulfilled are those interests which do not satisfy the person's needs and desires. Individuals will frequently report that these interests do not provide a sense of pleasure and they will often complain of having underlying difficulties with decreased motivation and follow-through

Upon recognition of personal needs, the objective becomes the clarification of characteristics of activities or interests which coincide with the person's needs. The therapist needs to explore supportively and parallel the person's use of time, and patterns of behaviour observed in the setting. The therapist can help to identify barriers which inhibit follow-through or interfere with the individual's sense of satisfaction with the activity. Another therapeutic idea is to maintain an ongoing discussion of how individuals structure and use their leisure time outside the setting. Is the person able to follow through expressed desires and leisure goals? Are there barriers or underlying problem areas present which inhibit follow-through with personal goals? Upon identification and awareness of the problem areas, the therapist can facilitate exploration of alternatives and constructive ways of dealing with obstacles.

Many individuals will participate and report on enjoying the activities presented in the programme. Some will request to take their projects home to work on during their leisure. It is recommended in day-treatment that the therapist encourage the person independently to pursue and obtain a similar project using resources in the community. If the therapist provides projects to structure their leisure outside the setting, this diminishes the opportunity for individuals to explore community resources and become skilled at meeting their own needs. The therapeutic objective is to encourage individuals to become aware of their needs and explore ways in which they can meet them independently.

Identification and Constructive Coping with Emotions

Individuals who identify with this problem area generally report having difficulties with the identification of feelings. In addition, they like to improve their ability to cope with emotions. Improving identification of feelings refers to increasing one's awareness, understanding and ability to recognize emotions. When individuals identify the desire to cope more constructively, they are referring to increasing their ability to adjust, adapt and successfully handle emotions without being overwhelmed. Coping mechanisms are both the conscious and unconscious ways people adjust to emotions and environmental demands without altering their goals or purposes.

The therapeutic issues focus on the expression of feelings and recognition of associated behaviours of the problem area. Helping the individual to parallel observed behavioural changes with their internal, emotional experience while in the setting can be helpful in increasing awareness and developing new ways of coping. To assist with improving a person's coping abilities it is helpful to identify the characteristic ways in which they respond to emotions and to identify barriers which interfere with their constructive handling. For individuals to be able to channel emotions constructively, they need to become aware of their personal control. There are advantages and disadvantages to the many ways of expressing emotions and these need to be explored.

Matching appropriate activities with the individual's needs and emotional level can also facilitate awareness, understanding and utilization of constructive coping strategies. For example, when an individual persists at a tedious, frustrating activity during a period of increased stress, the project may contribute to the person's increased anxiety and inability to function. Depending on the individual's needs and treatment goals, the therapist may encourage exploration of the person's emotional needs, coping strategies and utilization of activity. The treatment plan can be advised accordingly, when therapeutically indicated, to meet the individual's needs and provide a constructive channeling of emotions.

Frequently adjustments to the treatment plan are contra-indicated. An example might be when the primary goal is to learn how to cope and tolerate periods of increased frustration. The therapist needs to support expression of feelings, assist in recognizing behavioural patterns, explore options and clarify constructive alternatives.

Impulsive Behaviours

Impulsive individuals are those who have a tendency to act suddenly upon receiving a stimulus. The factors which precipitate an impulsive reaction are varied and differ from one person to the next. Often the stimulus is an internal experience such as thoughts, ideas or feelings. External factors may lie with other people or events within the environment. The distinction between impulsive behaviours and other kinds of behaviours is the urgency which demands immediate action. This urgency can be displayed in the manner in which people speak, make decisions or get things done.

The therapeutic idea when dealing with decreased impulse control is to explore and discuss the problem areas as they relate to issues of self-esteem, personal satisfaction, frustration tolerance and coping abilities. The therapist can increase awareness of the problem area as it is exhibited in the setting and assist in exploring alternative ways of coping or dealing with the underlying areas of difficulty. Supportive confrontation and clarification of the individual's decision-making process can be helpful to decrease impulsiveness and facilitate decisions based on one's desires and needs. When dealing with decreased frustration tolerance, the therapist needs to provide support, encourage expression of feelings and explore constructive ways of handling the situation as opposed to ways which the individual will regret at a later time.

Seeking Assistance

When individuals identify seeking of assistance as a problem area, they are generally referring to their experienced emotional difficulties along with a prolonged delay or hesitation before trying to get any help. They frequently will state that any attempt to ask for assistance remains difficult and creates a tremendous amount of anxiety and discomfort. For many the significance of seeking assistance focuses on the realization that difficulties experienced are outside the person's control. At this point they acknowledge that outside help is needed to overcome their experienced difficulties and assist with problem-solving and making things better.

The treatment ideas when working with this problem area are to assist individuals in recognizing associated behaviours, and increase awareness of the underlying issues regarding their style of seeking assistance. It is advisable to explore ways in which the person can challenge their difficulties and identify individual treatment goals of seeking assistance during the activity session. Some individuals may be encouraged to assert their need for assistance while others may be encouraged to ask for ideas or request information when attempting to solve problems independently. The therapist needs to modify her therapeutic approach respectively to facilitate the opportunity for individuals to work on their problem areas and encourage ongoing expression of the person's feelings.

Attention, Concentration and Organization

When individuals identify that they would like to be more organized and improve their ability to attend and concentrate, they are referring to limitations in their cognitive abilities and capacity to focus and organize their mental energies. When concentration and attention are the primary problems, individuals have difficulties focusing their thoughts and efforts in one area while at the same time excluding other thoughts and emotions from interfering. When the person's organizational abilities are limited, they are unable to arrange or structure their thoughts and actions in a meaningful or purposeful order.

If the individual's cognitive limitations are a result of an organic impairment, the therapeutic approach would be to provide a supportive, successful and structured experience to maximize the person's level of functioning. When the problem area is reflective and symptomatic of the person's emotional difficulties, it is advisable to explore the limitations as they are displayed during the activity setting and encourage expression of feelings. It is helpful to measure any relevant baseline data in order to assist in acknowledging any improvements or changes which will occur. The therapist may recommend projects which provide structure, successful experiences and remain compatible with the person's current level of functioning.

I Would Like to . . .

Providing an opportunity where the individual can write down a personal goal has proven to be the most interesting. The majority of independently selected goals appear to fall into two areas of concern. Individuals are either vague and unclear regarding problem areas and psychiatric treatment goals or they personalize their treatment goal in a manner which represents the individual's problem areas as unique situations compared to others. Both areas of concern represent underlying difficulties with resistance, acceptance of the patient's role and limited psychiatric understanding.

When individuals are vague regarding their problem areas and treatment goals, they may identify the desire to get better, overcome anxiety or be able to return to their place of employment. In this instance there appears to be a lack of awareness, understanding or personal responsibility regarding experienced problems and treatment goals. An example of when individuals identify their problem areas as unique situations may coincide with statements of wanting to overcome periods of binge eating or learn to live with a spouse's episodes of substance abuse. When dealing with these individuals, therapists often evaluate the person's behaviours as intellectualized, defensive and resistant to exploration of feelings. They may avoid discussion of painful topics or even deny that they exist. Frequently individuals will ask many questions, requesting specific answers from staff regarding how their problem areas will be addressed within the programme. These individuals can feel very threatened in the programme and many times choose to sabotage treatment or not continue with the programme.

The therapeutic idea here is to facilitate a supportive approach with the person so that a trusting relationship can occur. This is based on the notion that the individuals are able to make any gains in the areas of increasing their awareness, understanding and insight into their emotional areas of difficulty.

Conclusions

The detailed explanation of the patients' selected goals and problem areas forms the basis of the OT's principles in practice. The principles of practice specified in each problem area will help to solidify the therapeutic approach and psychiatric understanding required best to meet the needs of the day-hospital setting. Throughout this chapter reference has been made to individuals participating in individual craft or activity sessions. This form of practice has been very beneficial in day-treatment and remains a significant therapeutic aspect of the programme. Although group activities were not mentioned, they are also part of the day-treatment programme. Utilization of the patient-selected treatment goals and problem areas can also be applied to group activities.

The OT must have a high degree of psychiatric understanding, self-awareness and professionalism to treat this complex and higher functioning patient population. The behaviours exhibited within this setting are often referred to as subtle psychiatric signs and require experienced staff to deal effectively with them. The OT's assessment and evaluation of the patient's functional ability are most informative to the multidisciplinary treatment team. Occupational therapy's emphasis centres on action-oriented participation, where other parts of the programme emphasize verbalization skills.

References

DUNNIN, R.E. (1973) 'The occupational therapist as counselor', *American Journal of Occupational Therapy*, 27, 475–6.

FIDLER, G.S. and FIDLER, J.W. (1978) 'Doing and becoming: Purposeful action and self-actualization', *American Journal of Occupational Therapy*, 32, 306–7.

FIDLER, G.S. (1981) 'From crafts to competence', *American Journal of Occupational Therapy*, 35, 570–1.

Chapter 5

Rehabilitation of Long-Term Mentally Handicapped in Community Housing

Jenny Bodenham

In recent years there has been a recognition that people with a mental handicap are entitled to be given equal rights, dignity and respect. Old myths and superstitions regarding these people are still very prevalent — even amongst professionals, and some staff are reluctant to 'allow' a freer mode of life. Many of the handicapped people have accepted the restrictive enforcements of past years and find it difficult to realize their own potential and the opportunities now open to them. Therapists working in this field can develop a wealth of expertise, and revise and expand former knowledge; they can work as part of a multidisciplinary team and approach the major task of assessment and training with a wide range of participants of varied ages, cultures and abilities.

Some people with a mental handicap have congenital physical handicaps and others the physical limitations and impairments which come with ageing. Nevertheless, physical disabilities and communicative problems do not exclude people from rehabilitation programmes. Since 1976 our unit has undertaken various assessments and training modules catering for a wide variety of people. In the initial stages this involved people who were able to achieve a high level of independence in all aspects of daily living, and in more recent times our Health Authority has adopted a policy of gradual integration into the community for all residents. Obviously training programmes have to be relevant to the individual concerned, and to the type of accommodation and staffing offered.

Normalization, now professionally accepted, is still publicly a rather controversial area. Moving house or changing lifestyles is a major trauma to anyone, and people with a mental handicap are no exception; any public opposition can add to pressure on the mentally handicapped. Our work is expanding and necessitates the therapist being teacher, advisor, counsellor and friend; a model of guidance and support to the people who are being given these new opportunities. One needs to build up a good rapport to strengthen the person's confidence and identity. Stimulating the necessary motivation is a vital factor for success.

The Setting

Hanham Hall Hospital now caters for 186 adults and was modernized in 1983. A pilot assessment and training project was undertaken with the twelve residents, none of whom had much insight as to what living in the community would mean. This pilot scheme laid solid foundations for the work which was subsequently undertaken. Five moved to live independently in the house with little support from hospital staff.

In 1978 a major assessment and training module programme was undertaken to select suitable and interested residents to be given an opportunity to experience a totally different way of life. This was in semi-independent accommodation named Priory Court, which provided thirty places. These would require a very high degree of independence in all aspects of daily living including cooking, shopping, housework, laundry, and generally surviving with minimal supervision from a warden and other community services. Hanham Hall's therapeutic team devised a realistic and suitable training and assessment programme with constructive aims. The time schedule was eighteen months. An additional budget was provided to cope with the demands of the project. Training facilities were installed in the form of an OT kitchen plus a 'portacabin' to sleep two people, which provided a further kitchen, sitting room and bathroom facilities. Resources were limited, and staff and residents had much to learn about what was involved.

At that time there were few guidelines for such a venture and a lack of commercially available teaching aids. The OTs involved devised their own resource material and a separate manual is being evolved as the work is continuing with a wide variety of people, each of whom have their own requirements and the limitations imposed by their mental handicap. In view of the diversity of ability a programme must be arranged which can be presented in a variety of ways to stimulate motivation, facilitate enjoyment and achieve success for the participants. One must also remember that they are adults, albeit with special needs, who wish to be treated with respect. Priory Court training provided a survival programme; initially training in certain areas had to be rather low-key mainly because of lack of time and the risk of 'overload' of information to residents. Additional training sessions were undertaken after their discharge and a back-up community service team still provides for specific individual requirements. Originally seventy residents were shortlisted for this programme. Thirty-three were formally assessed and in 1980 seventeen were discharged durings its first few weeks. There was no pressure to fill the places as it is vital to avoid inappropriate placements. To date no one has been re-admitted or has asked to return to the hospital. Of the people who did not complete the course, some chose to quit because too much was involved or because it would involve separation from their friends.

Assessment

Subsequent programmes have followed a similar procedure. A basic assessment form (see Table 5.1) is completed for all participants — some are inpatients and some attend a day-house run by the unit which covers all aspects of living and provides opportunities for residential stays in the cabin, giving tangible experience of life away from 'home territory'. All areas of the form are completed and individual requirements can receive specific treatment. The basic structured programme and teaching methods are tailored to suit each participant's needs, and are kept flexible.

Project management relies on high professional standards of competence and integrity, and all disciplines must work towards a thorough, cohesive assessment. A certain degree of staff training and agreement on principles of normalization, assessment criteria and 'emergency' situation policies were formalized in the early stages of the project. In our initial work past histories were available on many of the participants. One must be careful not to influence one's judgment; each assessment must be given equal opportunity.

Assessment is an ongoing process and one must observe, either directly or from a distance, and record and evaluate the findings. Reappraisal of therapeutic objectives at periodic multidisciplinary conferences keeps one's goals on target, as planning of short- and long-term objectives is an essential part of professional treatment.

The Hanham Hall assessment form was devised and has been updated by a multidisciplinary team. The front sheet is a personal/factual data sheet, noting health and physical disabilities, medication, etc., followed by a list of aims relevant to all participants. Areas requiring special attention are asterisked or underlined and the following topics receive a page of questions with gradings of none/little independence, some independence, fairly independent or fully independent on such topics as self-awareness, behaviour, social adjustment, sexual behaviour, communication skills, preferences and interests, mobility, personal care, housecraft, safety and first

Table 5.1. Residential Assessment in Occupational Therapy 'Cabin' Projects.

Introduction to: Portacabin project/community home Safety in the home Fire precations	
Introduction to: Cooking Use of utensils Preparation of food Sequence of cooking	use of toaster, sandwich maker, microwave oven, gas/electric ovens
Types of shop Shopping Cleaning flat Use and care of vacuum cleaner use of bucket and mop	Budgetting Cleaning sinks Cleaning cooker Cleaning fridge/freezer
Bath — running of Cutting nails	Washing hair Cleaning bath/toilet
Cleaning shoes	Size of clothes
Green Cross Code	Use of bus
Use of cafe Use of telephone	Use of Post Office Use of bank
Use of launderette Ironing	Hand washing
Sewing on button	Sewing tear
Reading Writing	Time Money
First Aid	Emergency procedure
Assessment form Leisure activities in the home in the community	Sex and social education
Holidays — ideas of and how to plan	

aid, academic abilities (reading, writing, time, money, community living skills, use of telephone, etc.), use of community resources and employment. There is a facility to review each sheet at a later date.

Assessment forms can be voluminous and time consuming and are not necessarily productive. Therefore, one must decide which method will suit the purpose most efficiently and effectively. Assessments are made to aid decisions about the level of service which a person requires, identifying specific needs and assisting in short- and long-term programme planning. Implementation of structured programmes relies upon staff being conscientious and enthusiastic. One may have to be prepared for some staff reluctance to adopt new approaches of care and treatment. Motivation is vital from all — not just the resident!

Training

The main aims are to offer each person the opportunity to realize and achieve their maximum potential and capabilities through the following ways:

1 to develop latent skills and aptitudes through individual work or work in small groups which will assist in a more purposeful, independent and interesting life for these people within their physical and mental abilities;
2 to encourage pride in appearance, good posture and good standard of hygiene;
3 to encourage language development and communication skills;
4 to channel excess energy into purposeful activity and provide exercise of the whole body for physical and mental well-being;
5 to teach and improve standards of socially acceptable behaviour, tolerance and respect for others and increased awareness of the environment; to encourage contact with public facilities in the community;
6 to teach and consolidate specific skills related to activities of daily living as appropriate to the individual: mobility, Green Cross Code (road safety), money handling, time, reading, writing and housecraft.

When putting principles into practice the first person to assess is oneself! One should refresh and update one's knowledge, particularly of basic teaching techniques, and it is vital to allow time to plan a basic teaching programme. While few of us have ideal textbook conditions in which to work, one should bear in mind a few rules.

Teaching and learning are complementary processes influenced by individual needs, the needs of others and the place of action. Consider environmental factors, comfort, positioning, lighting, length of session, rest periods and the compatibility of companions. Provide a secure consistent environment conducive to learning.

Allow sufficient time. Make good rapport with the individual and gain their confidence so that they will participate. Define targets and be aware of present capabilities and behavioural characteristics. Provide realistic aims and treatment and be aware of limitations. Allow for learning in easy stages, increasing gradually in complexity, and allow the participant to proceed at their own pace. If working in a group, plan an activity to suit the whole group so that no member becomes isolated or bored and no member is in contention with another. Ensure correct learning of a task first; choose an appropriate method for teaching the skill. The range of options is increasing, but ensure that the training medium chosen enables learning to be directly related to practice and does not involve translation or change in logic. Task components should be taught separately in the correct sequence. Emphasis must be on accuracy rather than speed, and each procedure should be undertaken in manageable steps so that the individual is not taxed beyond their capabilities. Avoid despondency and failure. Much of our work involves demonstration; have everything ready with all equipment in good working order. Have a finished product ready if possible. Position yourself so that all members can see. Demonstrate slowly and 'briefly' and verbalize as each part is undertaken; be clear and give sufficient detail but avoid padding as this may detract from the main theme or cause overload of instructions. If possible, have the participants explain what you have done. Discuss any safety aspects and, if necessary, repeat the sequence and then the participants can practise. If there are several in the group, each one can have a turn. If the task is very involved, a one-to-one session is preferable. Our sessions often took the form of a group demonstration, and then an individual practice session followed directly. Most group members were tolerant of the wait or undertook a task with which they could cope unsupervised. Do not assume that they will be able to do a task automatically. It may be necessary to repeat the instructions several times, but do allow time for instructions to be understood. Many ordinary tasks, e.g., dressing, washing and feeding, may take a considerable time; the more complex the task, the more time consuming it will be. When you feel that the person is on the right track, gradually withdraw and supervise from a 'distance'.

The choice of teaching technique can be crucial. One must know one's resources and, of course, oneself. Visual aids have proved very successful and, if the therapist is able to provide spontaneous drawings emphasizing the topic, this is helpful. However, not all of us are artists and we must rely on pictures from magazines, suitable wall charts, books and posters. Project books for participants have been useful when a topic has been covered. Guidelines or reminders have been set out in such a way that the participant can refer to the folder and, hopefully, the information will jog his memory. Project material is often specifically made by the therapists and now we have wide resources of our own to call upon for subsequent work. Most sessions have a 'feedback' time and are given a follow-up discussion. Many quizzes and table games provide revision and many have enjoyed the fun element of a quiz (sometimes done on a similar format to popular TV games, and with which the learners can identify). Care must be taken with the choice of questions, suitably geared to encourage participation, and care must be taken not to demoralize with failure.

When planning a session, I have found it more successful if only one or two teaching mediums are used. One can be 'over-enthusiastic' about putting over a topic and all that results is a sheer muddle of ideas and a clutter of materials and equipment. Simulation/role play is very suitable for certain aspects of assessment, but is time consuming and requires confident staff who are not averse to putting themselves into 'set-up' situations. One must also be aware of unexpected events as something may trigger-off an unpleasant or unusual event.

One must use one's resources to the best advantage and call upon other agencies for help. Local Authority Education Centres (or equivalents in other countries) may have relevant leaflets, videos, slides, etc. which can be hired (often free of charge) and cover various everyday topics like self-care social behaviour and safety in the home. One can arrange for appropriate speakers from outside to come and talk to the group e.g., the local police on road safety and personal safety. Living in the community, residents will need to be aware of the local doctor, dentist, chiropodist, etc. Topics such as sex and social education may best be covered by a specialist teacher. Some staff may not be sufficiently confident to teach this sensitive subject and others may not be able to convey the information in a satisfactory way. Our project chose to hire the services of a professional teacher from the Brook Family Planning Service. I attended the sessions with the residents and have been able to take several follow-up groups with the initial members and their candidates.

Of course, there are always constraints on therapy e.g., the cost or time involved, and it is worth mentioning that our initial work was undertaken on a very limited budget. Over the years we have added to our resources, but expensive equipment does not guarantee success and one can lose one's direction of purpose and become enveloped in technology.

During our initial assessments, compatible pairs shared several residential stays of a fortnight in our cabin, taking into consideration their usual work programme. Each person usually was granted absence from work during residential assessments and was given an outline of what would be expected. A basic day's routine was followed, allowing for two specific project sessions per day.

Occupational therapy staff gave supervision from 7.00 a.m. until 7.00 p.m. and later if necessary! Abilities varied between groups, but usually one was able to compensate for another. Does it really matter if every person does not acquire every skill? Effects of long-term institutionalization were often evident. Many were able but reluctant to use initiative and waited for staff direction. Many needed specific directions before taking initiatives, and for many it was necessary to be specific in order to give them security, not because they were incapable. For many decisions were difficult because they did not know what the options were and in many cases it would have been too confusing to list all the available options.

Once the participants are enmeshed in unfamiliar situations one must watch for signs of stress. Stress manifests itself in many ways and may cause anger, resentment and inappropriate behaviour or violation of house rules. Avoidance is a typical response too. In stressful situations one must be aware that sheer overload of tasks and responsibilities can cause stress, and something which may be regarded as trivial or simple may not be thought so by the very inexperienced person. One must also regard outside factors as being very influential on the candidate/participant, e.g., goading from residents not on the training programme, and interruptions of friendships.

On return to the ward setting newly acquired knowledge may not be allowed to be implemented; simple examples of this may be making a cup of tea or a snack meal, or ironing personal laundry. Sometimes this is inevitable because of the ward set-up but sometimes (maybe due to internal politics) the resident might be denied access to facilities or be discouraged as it makes additional work. This may cause unnecessary strain on the resident. All staff should be aware of the training programme and resident's progress.

During the Priory Court training, instruction and supervision in all areas of housecraft were given. This section required very close supervision initially but most participants coped well. On subsequent visits many had devised their own routine and were encouraged to work with minimal supervision, gradually taking over responsibility for themselves. Great emphasis in this 'survival' training had to be placed on the planning of meals, shopping for and preparation of food. A weekly repeating menu (the content of which was checked by the dietician) was devised to provide varied 'straightforward' meals. Menus and shopping lists were illustrated with pictures as well as words to cater for the varying abilities and to encourage self-help in shops. The initial shopping trips were, for some, a traumatic experience, but they soon became familiar with tasks and gained confidence. Budgetting and general handling of money were, and remained for many, areas which required long-term supervision. The weekly allocation of money did not allow for mistakes or frivolities. There were several incidents of money being mis-spent or 'acquired' but as time went on this temptation subsided.

Cooking ability varied but most achieved a presentable result. Initially supervision was always available for main meals and a process of 'back chaining' applied; being there was often sufficient reassurance. Judgment regarding quantities to purchase and prepare proved very difficult and the sequence of cooking and timing showed lack of forethought and judgment especially when several items were involved, but most became quite competent and safe, although seldom challenging the choice of menu and being content to follow the set menu.

Problem areas did arise with personal care and hygiene activities. Prior to the rehabilitation programme men had not run their own baths and because of hospital routine were instructed when to change their clothing, have a bath, etc. Difficulties with shaving and cutting nails were common, and when unsupervised some did not change their underwear.

Many improved their handling of money, use of telephone and writing or copying their signature in an acceptable way (necessary for signing allowance books). The concept of timing proved very difficult even for those who could tell the time. Programme charts showing a clock face were followed with the use of a clock to play a sort of 'snap'.

Prior to discharge the residents met the community doctor, dentist, policeman and other community agencies. During the first few weeks at Priory Court they were taken by the community nurse to the various surgeries to enrol and shown the procedure for being seen. A Department of Health and Social Security (DHSS) grant had been available to all those leaving the hospital to set up home, and this proved to be quite a mammoth task for the OT who had to calculate what items should be purchased by which member of the group in order to have spent the same allocation.

On arrival at Priory Court residents immediately had to cope with rent payments; each had signed a tenancy agreement in line with the Housing Association policies. Several residents attended Adult Training Centres or Sheltered Workshops and received a small wage plus Invalidity Benefit. Others were entitled to different DHSS allowances and a few were in open employment and paid accordingly. DHSS allowances proved a problem as they often arrived late or were inadequate. This was a new scheme and the DHSS did not appear to have the appropriate guidelines. Some residents were a little resentful that they had less spending money than when they were in hospital. The initial months proved difficult financially, as the residents had no savings to fall back on, but over the period they have been there some of these problems have disappeared.

A hospital placement was held for three months as a precaution in case anyone wanted to return — they did not. Again institutionalized tendencies were very evident at first. The sharing concept was difficult to comprehend, belongings were still put back in their boxes and then locked in the wardrobe, few trusted their possessions to be unlocked in a dressing-table. For some it was difficult to believe in the reality of discharge. Immediate support was given to candidates by the OT staff originally involved — the resident warden, community nurse and social worker.

In the initial stages some required prompting about personal hygiene but there were few problem areas. Budgetting required assistance and for some it is still needed (food, rent, TV rental, clothing, bus fares, planning for holidays, leisure and club activities .all had to be allowed for). At this time pocket-money was somewhere in the region of £3.00 per week, which limited personal habits (e.g., smoking and drinking) and left little money for leisure activities. First priority was always given to food and essential bills. Many residents chose to continue using the picture shopping lists and menu plans; few chose to use initiative and substitute other items, and some continued to purchase items which they did not need. The degree of progress depended on the individual. Those still using lists tended to be those who were originally reluctant to go shopping. After about six months residents were well settled and the majority were eager to do more advanced cookery so advanced cookery sessions were taken in the larger kitchen at Priory Court. The sessions aimed at a more varied diet using basic ingredients in different ways, and many of the residents have now made cooking something of a hobby.

The Worker's Education Association (WEA) held weekly sessions in conjunction with the hospital psychologist, the emphasis being on social norms. This group were pioneers in this area, and it was important for them to be socially acceptable to the general public and integrated into the community. Before discharge emphasis had been placed on this need, but it was difficult to reinforce within the hospital. Priory Court residents could attend the hospital social functions if they wished and many did in the initial months, but as they gained confidence they divorced themselves from hospital life. Some belong to the public library and the local Community Centre.

Thirty-three men were on these intensive training programmes and there were many sessions and notifications to all interested parties, together with the writing of reports and assessments. The specific training programme budget was constantly logged, specifically how the money was spent, projecting future needs and qualifying this with relevant data for additional staff input, etc. At that time clerical help was limited and no computer facilities were available to record data. As with much of our work one has to substantiate the need for a facility in order to achieve it and this may mean carrying out excessive amounts of work, which could be undertaken by a clerical assistant thus leaving the therapist time for specific involvements with training, talks to interested parties, e.g., medical students, student nurses and local community groups. The therapist must be a good public relations officer and is often the mediator between hospital and community.

Walters (1982) has documented the history of events leading to the construction of Priory Court and selection details of initial inhabitants. Priory Court has a resident warden, but it is not a hostel and does not conform to other warden supervised dwellings. It offers an opportunity for thirty people to lead a relatively normal life with support from professional community services when required (Struthers, 1983; Burden, 1983). Some tenants work in the local community, some attend Day Centres and many have become integrated into community facilities for their leisure interests, but opportunities exist at Priory Court for them to meet socially with other tenants.

Outcome

Articles and reviews were written by the various disciplines involved.One article by the social worker took the form of a consumer survey: 'What do you think of it so far?' (Passfield, 1983b). None resented the household chores, and most enjoyed the freedom of choice and were still realizing opportunities. Research undertaken by the project's psychologists makes the interesting comment that the people chose for the scheme may have been rejected by some professionals as they were fairly limited intellectually (mean IQ 40), certainly not young (mean age 48 years) and had had a long period (mean time 39 years) in hospital (Staite and Torpy, 1983). The successful candidates had significant self-direction and it was generally felt by the team that people needed to be fairly proficient in money and language skills to survive in the community for this high level of independent living.

Success criteria for Priory Court were also influenced by continuity of staff and support throughout the training. Initial participants were well-known by staff prior to assessment, and basic support and trust were already established. The training area was in a known locality and the local community already accepted the residents as the hospital had been there long before the local housing. The Health Council organized a public meeting and there were ample opportunity for people to air their views. As for the candidates themselves, they had chosen to 'apply' and were not forced into this training. Some started the course wanting to assess it for themselves and then opted to discontinue. No one was in competition with their peers and each were placed to suit their needs.

This venture has proved to be remarkably successful in spite of any problems and fears about its practicability during the early stages. It does seem to prove the need for similar wardened housing units. There are many patients all over the country who could be helped to live in the community instead of in hospitals, if similar schemes could be established to train and resettle them. The hospital has been helped by being able to discharge patients to Priory Court, and the patients have gained enormously in confidence and pleasure in their achievements and independence.

Residential assessments in the cabin are still undertaken, other long-stay residents are enjoying using its facilities and a full, slower-paced rehabilitation programme is being followed. However, the cabin facility is also available to people presently living in the community, be it in a hostel, group home or with their family. Many of these people attend our training unit once per week and work with a small group all of whom are seeking a fuller way of life. Each person has an individual programme but benefits from the support of companions as many are on unknown territory and apprehensive. The cabin programme is modified to suit the individual. The set menus are no longer followed as in the Priory Court assessment, although most choose to complete the first week's menu chart and then repeat it for subsequent weeks. This is helpful when they are preparing shopping lists and budgetting, etc., although those adept at writing may choose to change more often. As mentioned earlier, our Health Authority, in line with a government directive, had adopted the policy of 'gradual integration' into the community for all our residents. As therapists, we are involved in a long-term programme looking at all residents to assess their needs and potentials, offering them different options and opportunities to try for themselves many of the living skills which we take for granted.

A housing trust has been set up to secure suitable properties in the area and as each dwelling is found, suitable residents will take up a different life style, and each home will be different depending on the location and type of facility. All homes will be small, some will be fully staffed and others may work on a 'core and cluster' system. At present many small groups of four or five are seen by the OTs giving the idea of family and each group being selected for compatibility. All aspects of the assessment form are covered, the emphasis being placed on self-awareness, awareness and tolerance of others, socially acceptable behaviour, mobility, personal hygiene, preferences and interests. Depending on the individual, varying degrees of housecraft are undertaken, the most popular of which are laying the tables and washing up. Emphasis is not placed on meal preparation and cooking as this may be done by staff, although residents, if capable, are encouraged to help.

It is worth repeating here that one must maintain an open mind and remain impartial. Many residents have shown aptitudes hitherto unknown. The institutional lifestyle has never offered some of the ordinary tasks of life and when this opportunity has been presented the person has excelled. Sometimes their past behavioural record has left little to be desired, but with the small group approach many seem less frustrated and very little aggression (if any) is seen. Compatibility of group members will be vital for small group living. During the therapy sessions we have been able to organize suitable groupings which seem to gel well.

Within these small groups an informal atmosphere has evolved and this has led the way to more purposeful discussion amongst the residents. Each appears more relaxed and willing to enter into conversations, to try out new opportunities and challenges, and they are even more receptive to performance appraisal sessions. Being supportive does not mean being patronizing; it means creating an atmosphere in which the person can admit faults and knows that one will listen, understand but not necessarily approve. Whilst one must give praise where it is due and constantly encourage better endeavours, overpraising can confuse the situation.

It is envisaged that the community houses will be home for three to six people. As each residence becomes available, the staffing service levels will be confirmed and standardized procedures outlined. There is always the problem of whether to purchase the dwelling first and then find the occupants or have a list of people with their 'life requirements' known and then look for suitable property. At Hanham both options are being followed, as the numbers currently involved for discharge into the community mean that everyone is being assessed and their 'life requirements' are now more specifically outlined so that when properties become available residents can be matched to accommodation. The physical location of some dwellings would exclude certain people but be suitable for others. Some residents in wheelchairs would require suitable access, whilst some structural alterations and ramping could be provided. Not all properties lend themselves to satisfactory conversion, and great care is being taken not to make these dwellings obstrusive. The whole concept is for the discharged residents to blend with the general community and be accepted as normal members of society.

All staff are being asked to be objective and to consider what is in the person's best interests. As these small homes develop, some staff will be redeployed to provide home support services. Certainly the service to the mentally handicapped is expanding and changing and all disciplines are having to assess and evaluate the present services and where necessary plan and implement a new programme. Staff should consider effective implementation of treatment plans and all are aiming to give a supportive service to residents. One should not be swayed by age or physical impairments, but should consider the person and consult with them.

'In-house' training courses and local exhibitions are being held to educate and inform people of these current developments. Absence of knowledge and lack of understanding can create problems and efforts must be made to alleviate such situations preferably before they occur. A therapist and other members of the therapeutic team may find themselves acting as public relations officers, giving talks, lectures, etc. to schools and local organizations. It is vital that the whole team adopt the same standards of socially acceptable conduct and ensure that residents attain and maintain their standard whenever possible as sometimes 'the public' are looking for 'faults' (residents are often confused as they see 'unacceptable' behaviour displayed by members of the public). We are seeking a socially acceptable standard from our residents/clients so that even if the standard lapses, overall behaviour is still acceptable.

Conclusions

Dissolution of institutions will take a long while to happen. People with a mental handicap receive a very different type of service from that of similar people fifty years ago. Medical research is progressing and many conditions are now avoidable or treatable. People with a mental handicap will always be part of society. Our efforts at present are to make them better integrated members who have much to offer given the opportunity. How can one judge success of treatment? Has one achieved one's aims to strengthen the confidence of a person, increase their knowledge of self-help and worldly skills, and provide interesting programmes through which they will realize what life expects and has to offer? There will be computerized information data regarding future requirements, budgets, etc. It will be some while before factual information is available concerning our present work, but a quicker non-scientific way would be to ask the people themselves.

References

BURDEN, P. (1983) 'No place like home', *Mental Handicap,* 11, 96–7.
PASSFIELD, D. (1983a) 'What do you think of it so far? A survey of 20 residents at

Priory Court', *Mental Handicap,* 11, 97–9.

PASSFIELD, D. (1983b) 'I like it here' *The Bridge,* 9, January–February, Hanham Hall, Bristol, UK.

STAITE, S. and TORPHY, D.M. (1983) 'Critical variables governing the selection of mentally handicapped people for inclusion in a supported independent living scheme', *Mental Handicap,* 11, 94–5.

STRUTHERS, J. (1983) 'Special needs housing for mentally handicapped adults', *Parents Voice,* MENCAP.

WALTERS, R. (1982) 'Residential care for mentally handicapped people', *Proceedings of the 15th Spring Congress on Mental Retardation,* MENCAP.

Chapter 6

Child and Family Psychiatry

Gill Trafford and Sheila Boyd

The role of the OT in child and family psychiatry depends considerably on her own personality and previous experiences as well as the ethos of a particular unit. There will be opportunities to work within the areas of individual child therapy, group work with children and families. A variety of childhood disorders are seen in a child psychiatric unit, e.g., emotional problems, behavioural problems, childhood psychoses and autism. This chapter outlines areas of work available to the OT by focusing on assessment of the child, group therapy for children, family liaison and family therapy.

Assessment of the Child

The Atmosphere

The interview room or play room should be quiet, equipped with appropriate play materials, and furniture should be child-size with at least two chairs, one being used by the therapist. When the therapist meets with the child it is important that the reason for coming into the playroom be expressed in a language which the child will understand. It is important to let the child know why he/she is coming to the room, how long for, and that the toys/materials in the room are exclusively for the child's use. If, in the assessment period, more information is needed about further aspects of the child's life, it is important to be encouraging and sympathetic. A problem should only be talked about if the child indicates that it is acceptable to do so. If play is not revealing, it is useful to ask the child to paint a picture of a relevant topic, or relate a situation to someone else and follow this up by asking if this perhaps happens to them. The best criteria for the therapist to help gain a good rapport with the child will be to be gentle, sympathetic, non-judgmental and facilitative.

Points of Note during the Play Sessions

The quality of the parent(s)/child relationship (or with other people in the room) should be described. Points to note are verbal and non-verbal communication, and feelings of warmth and care. When the child leaves the parent(s), observation should be made of how the child separates.

Child's appearance. Is the child of normal size and weight? Does the child look cared for? Are the clothes suitable and age-appropriate? Are there signs of ill health or bruises? Are there any obvious tics or odd mannerisms? Does the child appear restless, overactive or easily distractable?

Child's mood. Is the child sad or happy, inhibited or disinhibited, relaxed or fearful, warm or cold? Is the mood appropriate to the situation?

Child's reaction to therapist. Is the child friendly or hostile and challenging? Does the child ask personal questions? What kind of feelings does the child engender within the therapist?

Child's inner thoughts and conversation. By listening to the child and asking sensitive questions one can discover if the child thinks clearly and logically, whether there are any bizarre thoughts, what the child is preoccupied with, whether the language is expressive and whether the child understands appropriate information.

Child's play. The child's play will indicate to the therapist issues present in his/her life. Points to note include: How long does an activity last; what is the content of the play; is the play symbolic, absorbing, destructive, regressive, creative?

Child's fantasies. Asking about the child's fantasies will give some further information to the assessment. Things to ask include: What are your three wishes; what do you dream about; what would you like to do when you grow up?

The assessment stage could last for one or more sessions. Gradually an overall picture of the child will emerge, leaving the therapist with feelings about how to proceed. Alternatives may be for the child to be seen in the family setting or with the mother, psychological testing to provide additional information about the child's development, or individual therapy. When considering individual therapy OTs will have their own way of working with the child. The following therapies are available for individual child work.

Analytic Therapy

This approach was developed by Klein (1932) and Anna Freud (1946) who differed in their approaches towards transference issues between child and therapist. Also Freud felt that psychoanalytic techniques had to be supplemented by educational measures, whereas Klein felt that purely psychoanalytic techniques should be used. Five years of training are required for child psychotherapists.

Non-directive Play Therapy

Based on Rogers' (1951) client-centred philosophy, this technique was developed by Axline (1969, 1971). Basically, whilst the therapist accepts the child's situation, he is free to express himself through play. Where possible, exposed emotions and attitudes are reflected back to the child by the therapist, thereby clarifying these for the child. Axline feels that the child has the capacity for self-direction and growth.

Directed Therapy

This means directing the session to offer a structure which may help a child to focus on past, present or future events. This is an area to use creative therapy including such activities as poetry, drama, story-telling and use of craft material.

The above examples give a brief introduction to styles of therapy used with children. Other therapies often emerge from the basic styles, and generally the therapist will develop a style based on her own experience, the ethos of the unit, the literature, supervision and the experience of others.

Play is an important part of a child's development. When a child is given a play situation, one can observe the child working out, trying out and testing situations which becomes important at a particular point in a child's life. By using play the therapist is therefore able to enter the child's 'inner world' and with the child explore feelings, conflicts, fantasies and thoughts. For example, 4-year-old 'David' was referred because of the behavioural problems at home. Subsequently it was learned that these problems related to the birth of a sister. In the play session David would spend most of his time with a doll family and doll's house, constantly playing around the theme of a baby challenging his own attention from his parents. This situation allowed the therapist to enter his 'inner world' and share his conflict. Another example of play situations consists of the therapist being asked to play the role of the child. 'Janet' was overwhelmed by school and demonstrated her anxieties by inabilities to work. In play sessions Janet insisted that the therapist played the pupil at school and be subjected to a series of educational scenes. Janet in her role of teacher and the therapist in the role of the pupil together worked out Janet's hidden anxieties about school and therefore what could help her to relax more and enjoy school.

Practical Considerations of Play Therapy

Toys for therapeutic play. The following toys should help in building up a relationship between the child and the therapist, allowing space for fantasy play, aggressive play and regressive play. Useful relationship-building toys include construction sets and games which are short and do not take over the session, such as 'pick up sticks' and 'skittles'. Fantasy/projective play may be facilitated with a doll's house, cooker with pots and pans, male and female dolls with clothes, doll's cot, domestic and wild animals (families are useful), telephone(s), models of houses, trees, cars, aeroplanes, fences, etc., ambulance with hospital set (useful if the child is in or has been in hospital), clay, plasticine or 'playdoh', paint, brushes, felt tips, crayons and paper, and puppets (a family of puppets plus a witch or dragon will be useful). Regressive play will be enhanced by sand, water, paint, clay ('messy play'), baby doll with feeding bottle, etc.

General Considerations

Basically the aims of treatment are the same for each child; namely, to improve optimally all areas of function and to make life as meaningful and fulfilling for them as possible. This is best achieved with close liaison with all team members to the extent that there is an overlap of roles. The family, particularly with mother, is included within this team. As her main treatment media the OT uses play. Initially the sessions are very free, the therapist providing a variety of toys, paints and drawing materials and allowing the child to choose his own activity. This period is very useful because: (a) the therapist and child become acquainted in a relaxed, free atmosphere; (b) the child's ability to persevere with a task may be observed; (c) imaginative versus ritualized and stylized play may be noted; (d) hand function may be assessed; (e) choice of toys may indicate developmental level; and (f) communication with the therapist (e.g., seeking praise) can be noted.

The mother's presence is invaluable in these early sessions as she can help overcome any initial problems, such as language difficulties or management problems. In addition, many young autistic children have difficulty in separating from their mother.

As treatment progresses from free play to more structured sessions, most of the child's difficulties become apparent. Because of the child's language and impairment he may only understand key words. It must be borne in mind that the complexities of language may result in confusion and a general 'switching off'.

Group Therapy for Children

This form of therapy was developed in the 1930s by Slavson (Slavson and Sciffer, 1975) and developed by Ginott (1965) amongst others. Group therapy has been shown to have considerable value in the treatment of emotionally disturbed children. Generally speaking the therapy will either be 'directed' (activity-orientated), in which the therapist provides structure, or 'non-directive', in which the children interact without any structure.

The following are important aims of group work: (a) to develop a feeling of trust between children and therapists — the element of trust is often lacking because of previous experiences; (b) to encourage interaction between the group, thereby fostering a feeling of cohesion and belongingness. Children who need to be referred to a group seem to have lost the idea of integrating and sharing with their peers and families. They are unable to communicate effectively and this produces inappropriate emotion. Subsequently they feel isolated and perhaps bullied by others. Helping them to feel part of a group will increase their desire to integrate and share; (c) to gain deeper awareness of oneself and others. Children may need help to understand how they are feeling towards themselves, their family, their peers and their environment; (d) to provide an outlet for anxiety and aggression. Children often come to the group full of energy and this can be linked to certain anxieties and tensions; (e) to address and work through real life problems; (f) to allow the therapist(s) within the group an opportunity to enter the child's inner world, and clarify feelings and attitudes.

Communication and Language Disorders

Most communication with language disordered children benefits from them being involved in small group therapy. Ideally these would be groups of three or four children with two or three therapists. The children should be carefully chosen so that each one would gain from the other group members. They should also be of a similar developmental stage. The OT might choose a psychologist, speech therapist or teacher as co-therapists. Particular aims of this group of children include: (a) to promote social awareness; (b) to increase attention span; (c) to promote sharing and turn-taking; (d) to provide situations for initiating positive behaviour; and (e) for children to learn 'how to get on with one another' with the help of therapists. Activities include: (a) outings — to park, zoo, airport; (b) playing games — pass the parcel, musical chairs, musical bumps; (c) board games; (d) musical instruments; (e) art activities — as a group, making a frieze, collage; (f) constructing large jigsaws; (g) role play — in shops, in houses; (h) sand and water play; and (i) snack time.

All the above sounds very straightforward, but with the limitations that these children have the groups are more difficult than one might imagine. The therapist has to remain one step ahead of the children and be prepared to act very quickly. This is easier if the therapist has had the opportunity to get to know the child individually before the group situation is introduced. A free and natural approach is most suited to these children. The therapist must be flexible and amenable. If the programme planned for a particular day is obviously not going to work, it is best to change to some other activity rather than press on with that intended.

Family Contact

Parents are invaluable with advice on handling and managing their children. Children also need the security of knowing their position and close liaison between staff and parents ensures consistency of management. The families need to recognize that the therapist is there to support and advise them. This is particularly true in the cause of autistic children. When children are very young, again considering the autistic child, the mothers should be present at most treatment sessions. This will be necessary when there are separation difficulties between mother and child, and also because the mother may be able to help the therapist if problems arise in handling the child.

The parents provide vital information concerning the child and their management of the child. When taking a history from the parents, consideration should be given to the following areas: (a) presenting problems (e.g., when did it occur, precipitating factors, duration, effect, quality, any changes?); (b) personal child history (e.g., pregnancy, birth, infancy, developmental milestones, separations from mother?); (c) family and social history (e.g., mother and her own family, siblings, parental relationships, child-parental relationships, siblings' relationships with each other and parents, important life events?); (d) school (e.g., schools attended, consistency of attendance?); (e) peer relationships of child (e.g., clubs/groups, any friends, age and sex of friends?); (f) health and emotional state (e.g., recent illnesses, pain, activity, restlessness, tics, clumsiness, sleep pattern, eating, concentration, mood, habits and mannerisms?); and (g) sexual development (e.g., puberty, knowledge of?). From the detailed history will emerge relevant etiological factors and a greater understanding of the problem. If it is possible, the husband should be present at the interview. Not only would he be able to contribute to the history, but being present with his wife will give some indication of the quality of their relationship. Once the history is complete (this may take more than one session), appropriate intervention can then be taken. This may be individual child therapy, or referral for parent(s) to marital work or family therapy.

Family Therapy

Family therapy involves the treatment of the family group rather than treatment of an individual. This type of therapy has gradually developed in the last three or four decades when the families of psychiatrically ill patients were recognized as an important part of the referred patient world. Today family therapy is widespread throughout the USA, Canada, parts of Europe and elsewhere. It is certainly becoming a treatment of choice in many child psychiatry units.

A term which is often used within family therapy is the 'system approach'. This allows for consideration of the way the family functions, how members interact and communicate, how rules and boundaries are established and used, and who plays what role. General systems theory first developed when there was a need to bring together and create understanding of the classical sciences with the social sciences, and allowing a greater understanding of how the environment determined what happens to the parts within and allowing consideration of the whole. This has become a useful model for family therapists, allowing them to look at the functioning of the family as an entity rather than as a group of individuals. When a person in a family presents with a problem, all members are affected by this problem. For example, the therapist is interested not only in behavioural problems of a child, but also in how the behavioural problems are a result of or dependent upon the family's way of functioning. If there is room for change within the family, the therapist will be looking for suitable change.

Schools of Thought

It is important to look at some of the styles of working with families to illustrate what is available, but further reading would be necessary to create a greater understanding. Family therapists usually work within an open system thus allowing for input and output between members of the family system. If one considers this open system with a general systems approach, the following models are relevant: (a) the structural approach; (b) the strategic approach; and (c) the group analytic approach. Another more recent development is the behavioural approach, which will be mentioned briefly.

The structural approach. A prominent developer of this style is Minuchin (1974). A structural approach with families looks at the way change can be made within the family system by exploring boundaries, subsystems, the way in which families unite and the distribution of power from within. At times of crisis when the system becomes less flexible, abnormal patterns emerge and homeostasis prevents positive change. Therefore, by focusing and intensifying a subsystem change will begin to occur for the complete family system. The therapist joins in with the family's style of words and movements yet maintains a suitable distance to allow for encouraging change.

The strategic approach. Within strategic work (e.g., Haley, 1963; Selveni-Palazolli *et al.*, 1978) once again the subsystem is used to create change, but this is achieved by taking into account paradoxical communication, family myths and family rules. Often this is useful with exceptionally disturbed families. Interventions may take the form of strategy and create a new learning experience by considering the sequence of behaviour and alternative choices. The therapist maintains a professional distance from the family similar to an analytic stance, and often colleagues remain behind a screen as an aid to intervention.

The group analytic approach. This approach takes into account both the understanding of group analytic theory and the idea of systems theory. Skynner (1969), a pioneer in this approach, suggests three principles fundamental to the technique. The first is to re-establish the broken communication network. Secondly, is the establishment of an effective dominance hierarchy, allowing appropriate structure and control to be achieved in respect to the development stage. The third principle considers the development of the child as successive mastery of increasingly complex group situations, gaining assistance from parents or from the family therapist. The therapist working with the family consistently takes into account intrapsychic and developmental factors aiming to give insight to the family regarding how they function.

The behavioural approach. Those involved in this approach rely upon the observation of the family's behaviour, their work being based on facts rather than feelings and on observed events as criteria for intervention. The role of insight on the family's behalf is relegated from importance (see Chapter 8).

Most therapists develop their personal ideas from the various schools after their own experiences, education and with consideration of their unit personality type. However, it is important to have a framework to operate from and an understanding of family dynamics.

Some Practical Considerations in Family Therapy

The Family

The family is the most important institution in everyone's life. The term 'family' will evoke all manner of images and feelings for each person within its network. There is a whole range of feelings which emerge through family life, but whatever these feelings may be the family network remains an important feature in the lives of most people. Size and dynamics of families vary. The family in this society is considered to be the parents and children living together, although there may be extended members living within this unit adding further variations to the family. Even the family pet can have considerable implications within the family structure. It is important to recognize how our own view of the family can influence us when dealing with families.

Family therapy is concerned with all aspects of family life. The therapist must be aware of differences within family networks and be sensitive to a family's lifestyle. It is also important to recognize how one's own perception of the family could influence one's own approach to working with a family.

Phases of Family Work

When involved in family therapy the OT passes through certain stages. An assessment stage is necessary to identify how the family functions and to note the areas of malfunction. For example, there may be parents who do not relate to each other and the child seems to hold the power within the family. This stage may occupy one or more sessions. Whilst the assessment stage progresses, some commitment by the family should emerge. For instance, the child with all the power may be their focus in terms of seeing the therapist in the first place despite the therapist feeling a need to define the couple's marital issues. Once the assessment phase is reached and the therapist recognizes what to work with, she is able to make a contract with the family. Regular family meetings are then established and work progresses. Finally, comes the stage of closure, which is reached by positive changes occurring. However, closure can also occur because the family, for whatever reason, wishes to terminate their treatment, or because family therapy becomes an effective treatment for a particular family.

Pros and Cons of Family Therapy

Pros. This form of treatment is considered to be quicker and more effective than treating the individual. Because of the nature of the therapy several people are treated together; consequently it is less expensive. The process is based on the 'here-and-now' and therefore held to be more rational than some alternatives.

Cons. Collecting the whole family together may be a problem, and it is said that it fails to tackle intrapsychic pathology. The family as a whole may be difficult to engage and work with.

Conclusions

Family therapy is by no means a new technique and it continues to develop. There is evidence that it is a worthwhile form of treatment, but more research needs to be carried out to give it a more scientific foundation. There are various schools of thought to be considered by those interested in family therapy. This chapter on family therapy is no more than an introduction to the subject.

References

Axline, V.H. (1969) *Play Therapy,* New York, Ballantyne Books.
Axline, V.H. (1971) *Dibs: In Search of Self,* Harmondsworth, Penguin.
Freud, A. (1946) *The Psychoanalytic Treatment of Children,* London, Imago.
Ginott, H.G. (1965) *Group Psychotherapy with Children,* 2nd ed., London, Penguin.
Haley, J. (1963) *Strategies of Therapy,* New York, Grune and Stratton.

KLEIN, M. (1932) *The Psychoanalysis of Children,* London, Hogarth Press.
MINUCHIN, S. (1974) *Families and Family Therapy,* London, Hogarth Press.
ROGERS, C.R. (1951) *Client-centred Therapy,* Boston, Houghton Mifflin.
SELVINI-PALAZZOLI, M., CECCHIN, G., PRATA, G. and BOSCOLO, L. (1978) *Paradox and Counterparadox,* New York, Jason Aronson.
SKYNNER, A.C.R. (1969) 'Indications and contra-indications for conjoint family therapy', *International Journal of Social Psychiatry,* 15, 145–9.
SLAVSON, S.R. and SCIFFER, M.(1975) *Group Psychotherapies for Children,* New York, International Universities Press.

Chapter 7

Pediatric Occupational Therapy within a Cognitive-Behavioural Setting

Carolyn Hatje Kaufman, Rachel Davis Daniels, Patricia A.R. Laverdure, Robin Moyer and Laurie Campana

This chapter describes the role of the OT in treating emotionally and learning disabled children. The information is based on a developmental frame of reference with the premise that it is the role of the OT to address the developmentally relevant functional abilities of these children. Treatment approaches include sensorimotor, cognitive and social-emotional perspectives. Case material is based on children at the Joseph P. Kennedy Memorial Hospital for Children, Massachusetts, a pediatric rehabilitation facility. The case studies are based on children seen in the OT department, with certain aspects of information altered to maintain confidentially and provide educational examples. In each case the emphasis is placed on the domain of concern related to that particular age group. Therefore, each case study may vary slightly, but the underlying principles are the same. The children described are from the Cognitive-Behavioural Programme which consists of three developmentally-based units. Children are admitted to this particular hospital because they are unable to cope with the tasks of daily functioning due to developmental or learning deficits, physical injury or illness, or psychological and/or social disability. Through the use of activities, the OT provides a foundation for development and promotes optimal functioning.

The model of human occupation is the theoretical framework used to organize the role of the OT with these children (see Table 7.1). For additional information regarding this model see Bruce and Borg(1983) and Kielhofner (1983, 1985).

The model of human occupation is based on the premise that all human beings have an occupational nature. Occupation is defined as the productive behaviours found in work, play and self-care which originate from the innate urge to explore and master the environment. The second premise of the model is that human beings are open systems interacting with the

Table 7.1. Components of the Model of Human Occupation.

PERFORMANCE SUBSYSTEM
Skills
Communication/interaction
Process
Perceptual motor
Skill constituents
Symbolic
Neurological
Musculoskeletal
HABITUATION SUBSYSTEM
Roles
Perceived incumbency
Internalized expectations
Balance
Habits
Degree of organization
Social appropriateness
Flexibility/rigidity
VOLITION SUBSYSTEM
Personal causation
Belief in skill
Belief in efficacy of skill
Expectancy of success/failure
Internal/external locus of control
Values
Temporal orientation
Meaningfulness of activity
Occupational goals
Personal standards
Interests
Discrimination
Pattern
Potency

environment. An open system is a composition of interrelated structures organized into a coherent whole which interacts with the environment and is capable of maintaining or changing itself. In the model of human occupation the act of taking in information and processing it is called 'throughput' (Kielhofner, 1983). Throughput is conceptualized as a hierarchy of three subsystems: the volition subsystem, the habituation subsystem, the performance subsystem. The volition subsystem governs the overall system and is responsible for choosing and initiating occupational behaviours. The habituation subsystem organizes occupational behaviours into patterns and routines, with the performance subsystem responsible for producing occupational behaviour or actions. All of these subsystems comprise the open system of the child.

If one uses the model of human occupation with children, it becomes evident that each subsystem impacts upon the others two subsystems (Kielhofner, 1985). If therapy has an impact on the development of habits and routines of a child, the child will learn to have a sense of control and organization in his/her life which relates to the volition subsystem. It is important for the OT to consider all subsystems, and in so doing provide a holistic approach to treating the emotional learning disabled child. A case from each developmental stage will be presented including early childhood, latency age and pre-adolescence. While reading the case reports, bear in mind that the model of human occupation is the theoretical framework organizing a development approach to treating each child.

Case 1: Charlie

Background Information

Charlie was born a full-term infant following an unremarkable pre- and peri-natal course. Despite extensive developmental difficulties, Charlie had been able to cope in his environment until the age of $2\frac{1}{2}$. At that time the family was disrupted by parental separation and relocation. Following this disruption, Charlie developed behavioural changes. His appetite decreased, he became increasingly choosey about food, he began to have toileting problems, disturbances in sleeping patterns were noted, and frequency and duration of temper tantrums increased. At the age of 3 he was placed in a pre-school Headstart programme. Despite the structure and intervention provided, behavioural difficulties worsened. In addition, social skills deficits were apparent. Due to concerns over his behaviour and development, at the age of 3 years 4 months, Charlie was referred for admission and assessment at the Early Childhood Speciality within a Cognitive-Behavioural Rehabilitation Programme.

Evaluation Results

Performance subsystem. The following assessments were administered to evaluate the performance subsystem: Peabody Developmental Motor Scale, Fine Motor Subscale, Learning Accomplishment Profile, Fine Motor and Prewriting Subscales; The McCarthy Scales of Children's Abilities,

Perceptual Performance Scales and clinical observations. Charlie's movement skills were characterized by reduced proximal tone and stability. Automatic reactions of righting and equilibrium were delayed and he demonstrated a tendency to use protective extension responses. Reaching, grasping and releasing patterns were immature, and fine motor performance skills were equivalent to 24 months.

Charlie's responsiveness and discrimination of tactile and vestibular stimuli were impaired, resulting in a delay in the establishment of body percept and impaired motor planning abilities (Ayers, 1973). He presented with impaired temporal and sequential organization, which made it difficult for him to establish appropriate concept exploration skills (Heiniger and Randolph, 1981). His visuo-perceptual, perceptual-motor, problem-solving and symbol formation skills were delayed at the 18-month level. Little differentiation between himself and the environment made communication very difficult.

Habituation subsystems. The Vineland Adaptive Behaviour, Daily Living Skills Scales, along with observation and interview, were administered to evaluate the habituation subsystem. It was noted that Charlie showed poor development of habits and routines and had a disturbed sleep pattern. His understanding of time concepts related to daily routine was limited, resulting in very little organization of daily habits (Kielhofner, 1985). Charlie also demonstrated severely regressed toileting behaviours with overall self-care skill development ranging from the 18- to 24-month level.

Volition subsystems. Patient observation and interview were used to evaluate this subsystem. Charlie demonstrated a diffuse understanding of himself and the environment which significantly reduced his sense of his impact on the environment. He showed little automomy and control of events around him with an inability to delay gratification. Initially a limited response to behavioural interventions was noted due to his difficulty understanding his role in organizing his own behaviour.

Treatment Goals

The performance subsystems.

1 Improve development of skill constituents in areas of:
   (a) interpretation and integration of movement challenges,
   (b) fine motor performance,
   (c) body schema/perception.
2 Improve cognitive/adaptive skills.

3 Enhance visuo-perceptual and perceptual-motor skills.
4 Improve differentiation and modulation of response to sensory stimuli in order to enhance social communication and interaction.

The habituation subsystems.
1 Enhance routine behaviours for feeding, toileting, self-care, and peer interaction.
2 Enhance behavioural repertoire/differentiation to improve his role of player and explorer of the environment.

The volition subsystem.
1 Enhance sense of self as controlling own body and movement.
2 Develop a beginning sense of control and mastery of the environment.

Course of Treatment

Occupational therapy services were provided within a multidisciplinary team format with direct OT intervention provided in individual sessions, small group sessions and structured classroom settings. Therapeutic focus within the performance subsystem included gradual introduction of movement experiences and tactile exploration. A sensorimotor approach was utilized to establish cognitive and adaptive skills and perceptual motor skills. The combination of graded sensory experiences, environmental structure and behavioural and cognitive accommodation provided the foundation for improved responsiveness to sensory stimuli. This foundation enhanced the development of the habituation subsystem in terms of social interaction and communication. The volition subsystem was addressed during movement experiences by providing the opportunity to control movement. This allowed Charlie to master his environment and believe in the efficacy of his skills.

Treatment Outcomes

During his inpatient stay Charlie was seen for approximately six months prior to re-evaluation. He was re-evaluated using tools similar to those used when he was tested initially. During testing Charlie required structure and consistent cueing due to distractability and occasional overstimulation.

Performance subsystem. Charlie showed gains in postural and proximal stability through the improved ability to maintain static trunk positions. Improved equilibrium responses, righting reactions and decreased use of immature protective extensions were noted. These gains contributed to a significant improvement in Charlie's ability to integrate and interpret movement challenges. As a result Charlie frequently initiated activities involving moving surfaces, running, climbing and jumping off raised surfaces. The Peabody Developmental Fine Motor Scale indicated skills at a 38-month level, showing a significant gain of fifteen months. Particular gains were noted in the areas of grasp and release patterns, manipulation skills and eye/hand coordination. Improvements were noted in body part relationship perception with skills observed at the 3-year-6-month-level. Charlie was able to imitate simple motor patterns at a 3-year-level.

Clinical observation indicated significant gains in attending and organizational skills. When given structure and cues, Charlie could imitate and complete a task in a more organized manner while attending for ten to fifteen minutes. In the area of visual perception Charlie demonstrated skills at the 3-years-6-month-level indicating more than a 12-month gain since initial testing. Charlie's visual motor skills improved with a noted gain of more than twelve months. In social communication and interactional skills Charlie again showed improvements. Given a model and cues, he was able to develop the ability to verbalize his needs and his discomfort when overstimulated. He also demonstrated a developing ability to internalize these strategies and use them appropriately when interacting with his peers.

Habituation subsystem. Charlie's improvements in sensory processing and body awareness enhanced his participation in daily living activities. Given a consistent approach and structure, Charlie was able to begin participating in scheduled toileting and mealtimes. He began to participate actively in dressing, performing at a 3-year-6-month-level. He developed habits within a daily routine, which he began to anticipate. With improved integration and interpretation of himself and his environment, Charlie was able to begin successfully exploring activities and toys within his environment, resulting in independent solitary play skills and the emergence of parallel play.

Volition subsystem. During play Charlie developed a sense of being able to control his body movement in relation to the environment. He often initiated games involving the control and speed of movement. His improved ability to communicate verbally allowed him to perceive the impact of his actions on others. Charlie's developing ability to use coping strategies when overstimulated or in discomfort allowed him to gain greater control of the environment, while remaining in control of his responses.

Recommendations

During hospitalization Charlie benefited from OT on an individual and small group basis. Significant gains were realized in all developmental areas, and he demonstrated the ability to maintain and generalize acquired skills. OT was recommended to enhance his fine motor and perceptual motor skills. Consultation with his school teacher was recommended to develop his role as player and student.

Case 2: Brendan

Background information

Brendan, a 7-year-old male, was referred to OT during his admission to an inpatient cognitive-behavioural programme. Concerns regarding verbal aggression, difficult behaviour at home and school and academic difficulties were the impetus to his admission.

Brendan was the product of an uncomplicated pregnancy but with respiratory difficulties at delivery. His mother reported that his developmental milestones were achieved within normal limits. Behaviours described at school included verbal aggression, impulsiveness, distractability, difficulty conforming to class rules and a tendency to lie to teachers and peers. Brendan's mother was concerned about his behaviour at home. She felt that his difficulties stemmed from the inconsistencies of his father's presence in the home and the father's previous sexual abuse of the female children. The mother tended to deny Brendan's difficulties and instead blamed his sisters for problems that occurred. As a result, there was a high level of sibling animosity.

During his hospitalization Brendan participated in individual OT two or three times per week, as well as attending sessions in a class group and gross motor group. Treatment was coordinated with the multidisciplinary team via informal collaboration and regular attendance at team, unit and community meetings.

Evaluation Results

Performance subsystem. For all assessment areas Brendan's attentional problems were manifested by a high activity level with difficulty controlling his behaviour. The possible impact of medication on Brendan's attention was unknown as his family opposed such treatment. Intelligence testing by the psychologist revealed a discrepancy between his verbal and performance abilities in that whereas the performance score fell within the average range, his verbal score was significantly lower. Speech and language testing determined that Brendan's ability to discriminate auditory information was an area for concern and that there was a moderate to severe dyspraxia.

OT evaluation of his performance skills used the Southern California Sensory Integration Tests, the Bruiniks-Oseretsky Test of Motor Proficiency (Bilateral Coordination, Upper Limb Speed and Dexterity, and Visual Motor Control subtests), the Gardner Test of Visual Perceptual Skills, and the Beery Developmental Test of Motor Integration, as well as clinical observations. During OT assessment of his motor skills Brendan demonstrated generalized difficulty in organizing himself to perform unfamiliar gross and fine motor movements. Motor planning problems were particularly evident for bilateral tasks and appeared to be related to insufficient sensory feedback (i.e., tactile and proprioceptive) regarding the organization of his body scheme (Ayers, 1973). His discrimination of touch was impaired, with his left hand discriminating significantly more accurately than his right. Other asymmetries were noted, including primitive reflexes and posturing on the right but not on the left body side. Equilibrium responses were mildly depressed overall and somewhat more so on the right. Brendan displayed instability in his upper extremities and lacked a solid postural base for controlled motion with flexor muscle control less developed than extensor control (Bly, 1983). Brendan's perceptual skills were delayed by approximately one year. His disabilities reflected not only right visual field neglect but also his cursory attention to detail, limited figure/ground perception and impaired visuo-spatial relations. The effects of his perceptual deficits in conjunction with his motor planning difficulties were seen in his attempts to form letters, i.e., his difficulty discerning where to start and his use of unpredictable motor patterns.

Habituation subsystem. Interviews and review of Brendan's progress revealed that he was able to perform age appropriate self-care activities with supervision. An overprotective family which held low expectations for Brendan and blamed his siblings for problems deprived him of the opportunity to take responsibility for his behaviours and to define his role as a family member. Brendan's environment was loosely structured resulting in a poorly established sense of time. At home and at school Brendan was isolated from his peers as a result of stealing, fabricating stories and verbal aggression. Therefore, his role development as a friend was poorly established. In the student role Brendan benefited from external structure. However, in a large classroom he had difficulty in following rules and was unable to sit for five-minute intervals.

Volition subsystem. Comparison of results from the Piers-Harris Children's Self-Concept Scale and interview regarding perceived competence revealed similar profiles. All areas were below the normal range for age with social skills, popularity, behaviour and anxiety being more depressed than the physical appearance and cognitive areas. Review of psychological testing suggested a child who viewed the world as aggressive and himself as being damaged. He had a liability for associational, fantastic and disorganized thinking with suicidal ideations. In keeping with his view of himself as damaged, Brendan had difficulty with the risk involved in attempting difficult activities, accepting criticism and forming close attachments.

Brendan demonstrated interest in a variety of hobbies including construction activities, making card houses, forts and riding his bike. These activities reflected his areas of strength, including fine motor skills, dynamic balance and creativity, although they also increased his isolation from peers.

Treatment Goals

Performance subsystem

1 Maximize motor control via enhancing postural stability, equilibrium response, motor planning and bilateral integration.
2 Normalize sensitivity to touch and movement. Develop accurate tactile discrimination.
3 Improve organization of visual scanning.
4 Develop age-appropriate visual perceptual skills with emphasis on attention to visual detail, figure/ground perception, and visuo-spatial relations.
5 Develop a consistent approach to letter formation by using a predictable motor pattern and a top-to-bottom, left-to-right sequence.

Habituation subsystems.

1 Develop sense of time.
2 Improve ability to organize himself with reduced external structure.
3 Improve performance in the role of student.
4 Improve performance in the role of peer.

Volition subsystem.

1 Improve accuracy of self-concept incorporating knowledge of strengths and weaknesses.
2 Improve ability to involve peers in his play.
3 Improve self-esteem via opportunities for mastery of performance skills.

Course of Treatment

As Brendan was easily disorganized by visual or auditory stimuli, the treatment environment was structured for controlled addition of stimulation. In a small group it was helpful to have only one person provide verbal structure and directions. Eye contact was requested not only as Brendan neglected to look at people during interactions with them, but also because this resulted in a calmer behavioural state with decreased provocation. Brendan's creativity, enthusiasm and interest in constructional tasks were tapped as strengths to augment treatment.

Brendan's motor control was addressed by providing graded movement challenges which elicited greater postural control, more efficient equilibrium responses, increased bilateral integration and more mature rotational patterns (Bly, 1983). Control of flexor musculature and flexor holding patterns were emphasized to promote the development of praxis. Self-administered linear vestibular input was used to decrease oversensitivity to movement. Proprioceptive input involving heavy work and resistance normalized Brendan's sensitivity to light touch. Discriminative tactile experiences, tapping graphesthesia and stereognosis were engaged in as tolerated (Ayers, 1973). To enhance manipulative skills, stability of the shoulder, wrist and fingers was emphasized as well as activites to develop the arches of the hands (Bly, 1983). Cues were provided to facilitate organized scanning of perceptual tasks. Attention to visual detail, particularly when noting similarities versus differences, was also emphasized. Letter formation was reinforced in conjunction with Brendan's classroom teacher by providing cues regarding a starting point and teaching similarly formed letters as a group.

To develop more consistent habits, treatment was scheduled on a consistent and predictable basis, Brendan's personal schedule card was reviewed as needed in order to foster his sense of control over time. Structure and clear limits were provided to facilitate his development of internal controls and organization. Facilitation of Brendan's role as a student was accomplished by gradually increasing the duration of activities to improve the length of his attention. Prerequisites for academic skills were remediated as described under the performance subsystem. His role as a peer was addressed by providing treatment in individual and dyadic sessions and eventually small groups of three to four children. Initially constructional group projects were used as Brendan had good performance skills in this area and thus could concentrate on his social interactions. Adaptive social behaviours were encouraged via direct cues and modelling (Furman, 1980).

To foster Brendan's self-esteem by acknowledging that he was both worthy of acceptance and capable of meeting challenges, a supportive environment was provided by the therapist in conjunction with the treatment team and the therapeutic milieu. Treatment activities were graded to his developmental level to enable success and enhance his sense of mastery. In addition, his family was involved in treatment sessions so that they could reinforce his developmental gains and positively reward his efforts. Thus Brendan and his family could witness his strengths and his weaknesses and gain a more realistic base for their expectations of him.

Treatment Outcomes

Performance subsystem. Brendan's postural control and balance were notably improved. Primitive reflexes were integrated. His sensitivity to touch and movement was within normal limits. Although his coordination was improved, he continued to rely heavily on visual monitoring when performing non-habitual motor acts. This strategy was most evident during bilateral tasks when it was necessary for him to watch one hand and then the other, thereby prohibiting simultaneous bilateral motion. His upper limb speed and dexterity for unilateral tasks, however, were within age expectations. He developed more accurate manual discrimination (e.g., stereognosis and finger localization) although there was still a discrepancy as his left hand was more adept than his right. Yet he developed a right hand dominance. Brendan's perceptual skills were enhanced as evidenced by more organized visual scanning and mildly increased ability to concentrate in a minimally distracting environment. Testing revealed increased attention to visual detail. Relative weaknesses clustered in the area of spatial relations and visual closure which related to his problems with letter formation. Given more structure (e.g., dot cues regarding where to start) and repetition of the motor sequences, Brendan was forming letters in a more consistent manner.

Habituation subsystem. Brendan's role as a student improved as the frequency of spontaneous eye contact with the speaker increased. This improved his ability to attend during school and small group activities although a highly structured environment was still needed. As Brendan's internal control developed, with staff control he was able to experience more success in dyadic and small group activities, thus improving his role as a peer. Another indication of his evolving positive peer role was that other children would seek him out as a playmate. Anticipation of forthcoming treatment sessions and the activities indicated an internalization of a sense of time.

Volition subsystems. The results of the Piers-Harris Children's Concept Scale and interview regarding perceived competence demonstrated a more accurate awareness of his difficulties. Although the profiles were similar to those seen initially, they were within the normal range for age. Social skills, popularity, behaviour and anxiety continued to be areas of concern. As Brendan's self-esteem improved, he was able to begin taking risks during treatment. Brendan's self-esteem continued to need development as his ability to take risks during re-assessment was reflective of earlier behaviours.

Recommendations

Prior to discharge the treatment team collaborated with the community school to arrange a self-contained, highly structured and well integrated school programme. This was to include individual counselling, crisis intervention and family counselling as needed during the school day. Academic therapies including OT were provided in dyadic groups for continued work on Brendan's peer interactions. The need for regular consultation between the OT and the school teacher was stressed. Treatment recommendations for OT were to refine developing abilities and involvement in a small physical education class with emphasis on motor skill acquisition and play development.

Case 3: Travis

Background Information

Travis was a 10-year-old male who was referred for assessment and planning to OT during his admission to an inpatient cognitive-behavioural programme. There were long-standing concerns regarding his emotional/ behavioural adjustment and poor academic achievement in a special classroom for children with behavioural and learning difficulties. The impression was of a youngster with cerebral dysfunction and hyperactivity although the effects of an adverse environment also needed to be considered.

Birth and developmental milestones were unremarkable, but his mother described Travis as being overactive from early in life. The home environment was chaotic and there was a constant threat of physical violence. Both parents had been physically absued themselves as children and one had a history of drug and alcohol abuse. Behavioural problems were particularly notable after commencing a Headstart programme when stealing, aggression and an apparent attempt to set the home on fire were of concern. It is possible that Travis was not able to establish himself as having a positive impact on his environment; his environment not allowing development of normal habits and routines, and not assisting in the acquisition of performance skills. He responded by spending as much time as possible away from home and acting out at school.

Evaluation Results

Throughout testing Travis required frequent encouragement and occasional limit-setting to complete tasks. Behaviourally he was distractable and fidgety. His attitude reflected expectations of failure and was punctuated by frequent negative comments regarding his performance.

Performance subsystem. The following assessments were administered to assess the performance subsystem: Jebsen Test of Hand Function, Southern California Sensory Integration Test: Motor Accuracy, Gardner Test of Visual Perceptual Skills, Beery Developmental Test of Visual Motor Integration, and the Raven Matrices along with clinical observations. In the areas evaluated Travis displayed age-level performance in fine motor skills, gross motor skills and in sensorimotor skills. Weaknesses were apparent in visuo-perceptual skills, visual-motor skills and non-verbal problem-solving. These weaknesses were evident when he attempted to complete tasks that involved moderately complex visual representations (as in mathematics or geography). He also displayed difficulties with handwriting skills requiring both visual-motor and visuo-perceptual skills.

Habituation subsystem. Information related to Travis' habits and roles was obtained through clinical interview, review of his progress and the psychologist's interview with the parents. Travis reported having no responsibilities at home and having spent as much time as possible away from his home to avoid 'problems' there; he was able to complete daily activities such as basic hygiene and grooming, but the organization of daily routines was poor. Role development in the areas of family member, friend and student were all poorly established. The family had been living in a state of crisis which led to the deterioration of whatever family member role development had begun for Travis. He reported having no friends and spending the majority of his time alone. As previously described, Travis' performance skills were poor and led to an inability to learn at the rate of his classmates. In school his behaviour was out of control with spitting, swearing, stealing and refusing to do academic work.

Volitional subsystem. The volition subsystem was assessed through the Piers Harris Children's Self-Concept Scale, clinical interview and observation. In completing the Piers-Harris Scale, Travis scored below average in all areas except for physical appearance and attributes. His self-concept regarding his behaviour and his overall happiness and satisfaction were significantly depressed. Clinical observation and interview revealed a child who was easily frustrated and lacked perseverence. He often felt that he 'couldn't do anything', and he would give up a task if it challenged him. He took little responsibility for his actions, with most of his responses to questions regarding his sense of the current situation being 'I don't care' and 'It's not my fault'. This also displayed his lack of sense of control over what happened to him. When asked about his interests, his only responses were that he liked listening to music, watching TV and riding his bicycle. All such responses reflected his isolated lifestyle and minimal peer involvement.

Treatment Goals

Performance subsystem

1 Improve task skill organization.
2 Improve visuo-perceptual skills.
3 Improve visual-motor skills.
4 Improve cooperative work skills.

Habituation subsystem.

1 Develop an organized approach to completing daily routines.
2 Establish expectations for therapy routines including timeliness and expected behaviours.
3 Improve performance in the role of student.
4 Improve performance in the role of peer.

Volition subsystem.

1 Improve self-esteem through successful participation in individual and group therapy.
2 Provide an opportunity for Travis to control his environment within the content of an activity.
3 Develop interests to include social interests with peers.

Course of Treatment

Performance skills were addressed through successful completion of visuo-perceptual abilities, visual-graphic abilities and use of computer programmes. Task organization was addressed during group activities where

Travis had to follow specific directions and sequences.

The formation of routines and habits were addressed through providing Travis with a programme that outlined expectations for performance during individual and group therapy (Robinson, 1977). He was given rewards for timeliness, appropriate interaction with peers and for completing all expectations. As Travis' performance in this area improved he felt more comfortable in his role of student and peer. The family member role development was addressed in family therapy sessions with the psychologist.

Goals in the volition subsystem were obtained through success-oriented experiences and activities in all aspects of Travis' OT treatment. Through planning his therapy sessions with peers when given choices by the therapist, he was able to take some control. Exploration of various activities allowed for the development of social interests including cooking, group singing and dancing (Reilly, 1974; McKibbin and King, 1983).

Treatment Outcomes

Performance subsystems. Progress in the performance areas of visual perception, visual-motor integration and problem-solving as assessed through standardized testing was minimal. Of significance is the fact that Travis' performance in these areas when working on the computer was significantly higher. This suggested that his lowered test scores in these areas were more a result of his emotional state rather than cognitive ability. Travis made significant improvement in his ability to communicate effectively with his peers as well as maintain his self-control in group situations where his needs were not immediately met.

Habituation subsystems. Travis was able to establish daily routines for himself with supervision from staff. He became aware of expectations for therapy routines, but he could not always meet those expectations without therapist assistance. His role as student and friend improved with the ability to participate in dyadic and group activities, significant aspects of these two roles. He was no longer being removed from his classroom for disruptive behaviour and was able to persevere with school work that was challenging to him. With adult supervision he was able to structure his free time with a peer, participating in interactive activities.

Volition subsystems. The activities that Travis participated in, combined with his improved role performance, indicated an increased belief in his effectiveness within the world. He was finally feeling a sense of control over what was happening to him through developing his own sense of internal control. The activities which he learned during therapy sessions became interests for him and therefore allowed active participation with others and consequently less isolation. He continued to have concerns regarding his behaviour and overall happiness, but these concerns no longer dominated his thoughts and actions.

Recommendations

After six months of inpatient treatment the team felt that Travis was ready for discharge to a twenty-four-hour residential facility. Returning home was not an option due to the lack of support and supervision in the home. He had met the goals of his hospitalization and was no longer in need of inpatient hospitalization. Continued individual OT was not recommended, although he was recommended for pre-vocational training with an emphasis on functional handwriting, task completion, organizational skills, and to develop work skills and habits.

Conclusions

The three cases presented in this chapter are a sample of the type of children seen in a pediatric cognitive-behavioural unit. They represent the various developmental stages and disabilities that a therapist may encounter. At each developmental stage there is a slightly different emphasis for treatment. In the early childhood years the focus is on acquiring performance skills to provide a foundation for future growth and to allow for the development of occupational behaviours (Lindquist *et al.*, 1982a, 1982b). There is a strong emphasis placed upon the child's ability to interact with his/her environment and to make sense of those interactions (Kielhofner, 1985). During the middle childhood years there is a move away from the immediate environment and family to the school environment which includes the start of substantial peer interactions. It is during this time that the child should be mastering the basic skills of early childhood and beginning to concentrate on organizing those skills into habits and routines related to school and play. The later childhood years focus on refinement and expansion of all the previous mentioned areas. The child at this age should be developing the foundation for the exploration of future, formal occupational roles.

The model of human occupation is a hierarchical, open system model with all of the subsystems impacting on each other (Kielhofner, 1983). For this reason each subsystem is evaluated and addressed in therapy. It is necessary for the OT treating emotional learning disabled children to have a developmental perspective as well as an understanding of the subsystems described in the model of human occupation. Given the areas of concern for each developmental stage, it is not surprising that each case report varies in terms of which subsystem is more heavily emphasized. A developmental approach within the framework of the model of human occupation will provide the OT with a thorough understanding of her role within this population.

References

AYERS, A.J. (1973) *Sensory Integration and Learning Disorders,* Los Angeles, Calif., Western Psychological Services.

BLY, L. (1983) *The Components of Normal Movement during the First Year of Life,* New York, Neuro-Developmental Treatment Association.

BRUCE, M. and BORG, B. (1983) *Frames of Reference in Occupational Therapy,* Thorofare, N.J., Charles B. Slack.

FURMAN, W. (1980) 'Promoting social development', in LAHEY, B. and KAZDEN, A. (Eds), *Advances in Child Clinical Psychology,* London, Pergamon.

GREENSPAN, S. and LOURIE, R. (1981) 'Developmental structuralist approach to the classification of adaptive and pathological personality organizations: Infancy and early childhood', *American Journal of Psychiatry,* 138, 725–35.

GREENSPAN, S. and PORGES, S. (1984) 'Psychopathology in infancy and early childhood: Clinical perspectives on the organization of sensory and affective thematic experience', *Child Development,* 55, 49–70.

HEINIGER, M.C. and RANDOLPH, S.L. (1981) *Neurophysical Concepts of Human Behaviour,* St Louis, Mo., C.V. Mosby.

KIELHOFNER, G. (1983) *Health through Occupation: Theory and Practice in Occupational Therapy,* Philadelphia, Pa., F.A. Davis.

KIELHOFNER, G. (1985) *A Model of Human Occupation,* Baltimore, Md., Williams and Wilkins.

LINDQUIST, J.E., Mack, W and PARHAM, L.D. (1982a) 'A synthesis of occupational behaviour and sensory integrative concepts in theory and practice, Part 1: Theoretical foundations', *American Journal of Occupational Therapy,* 36, 365–74.

LINDQUIST, J.E., MACK, W. and PARHAM, L.D. (1982b) 'A synthesis of occupational behaviour and sensory integrative concepts in theory and practice, Part 2: Clinical applications', *American Journal of Occupational Therapy,* 36, 617–23.

MCKIBBIN, E. and KING, J. (1983) 'Activity group counseling for learning-disabled children with behaviour problems', *American Journal of Occupational Therapy,* 36, 433–7.

REILLY, M. (1974) *Play as Exploratory Learning,* Calif., Sage press.

ROBINSON, A.L. (1977) 'Play, the arena for acquisition of rules for competent behaviour', *American Journal of Occupational Therapy,* 31, 248–53.

Chapter 8

Occupational Therapy in a Behaviour Modification Setting

Gordon M. Giles and Donna Schell

This chapter describes the role of the OT within a token economy unit for behaviourally disturbed adolescents. Although the use of behaviour modification goes in and out of vogue, it has always been controversial (Edwards, 1982). Due to the interdependent nature of the treatment approach, it is not possible to discuss the effectiveness of OT in isolation. The chapter therefore concludes with a discussion of the general effectiveness of the unit with special reference to functional living skills.

The Geoffrey Hawkins Unit (GHU), which is described here, is a nineteen-bedded purpose-built ward located within the grounds of a psychiatric hospital. The central focus of the unit is upon patients who cannot live in the family setting or be treated as outpatients because of their frequent recourse to highly disruptive behaviour. The immediate and most pressing goal of intervention, therefore, is to help the individual gain some control over their inappropriate behaviour. Patients of either sex are accepted for treatment and are usually between 12 and 20 years of age. Most patients have a mild to moderate degree of mental impairment although occasionally patients of normal intelligence but who fulfil the other treatment criteria are admitted. Persons with major physical handicaps or severe organic deficits are not admitted.

The treatment team comprises a consultant psychiatrist, clinical psychologist, nursing staff, OT, remedial teachers, social worker, physical education instructor and dietician. A high level of efficiency in communication between nursing staff and the other disciplines within the treatment teams is essential if the token economy is to be applied consistently. Communication takes place at ward rounds, the hand-over periods between shifts which the OT attends, and at the weekly planning meetings where all disciplines plan activities for the week. The functioning of the behavioural programme and treatment methods used are reviewed briefly before examining the role of the OT in detail.

The Token Economy

The general principles of token economy systems are well known (Sheldon, 1982). Behaviour modification techniques have been used frequently with delinquent, mentally retarded, classroom and psychiatric populations. Reviews of programmes which look at outcome have shown them to be effective in producing behavioural change in these populations (Kazdin and Bootzin, 1972). For example, Cohen (1968) describes the use of token reinforcement with institutionalized delinquents in an attempt to develop academic skills. Individuals were not punished for not studying; however, points exchangeable for certain privileges were awarded for studying and task completion. After eight months most of the subjects had made substantial progress and the improvement was maintained on follow-up. A programme closer in orientation to that used on the GHU is described by Burchard (1967). The population treated were mildly retarded delinquent adolescents (IQ ranging from fifty to seventy). A general ward programme was developed which concentrated on reducing aggressive behaviour and developing skills. This treatment approach was shown to be effective on a number of measures using an ABAB research model.

The principles of operant conditioning indicate that learned behaviours are more likely to be repeated if they are followed by reinforcing consequences and less likely to be repeated if they are not. Bandura (1969) suggested that three components are essential to the use of reinforcement principles in the treatment setting. These are: (a) contingency of consequences, (b) an incentive system, and (c) a means of establishing appropriate behaviour. The system which operates on the GHU meets these criteria. The token system, which has been in use for a number of years, has been the result of a gradual development, attempting to meet the needs of a particular client population.

Tokens are awarded hourly and are dependent upon behaviour and performance within the programme for the previous time period. A record is kept of all earnings and failures to earn. The criteria for earning are adapted by the unit staff to the patient's level of functioning. Physical aggression, however, always results in failure to earn. Privileges are dependent upon token earnings. Complete meals require a certain number of tokens and not having the required number may result in earning only a part-meal (main course only). Should patients fail to earn tokens on two occasions within a twelve-hour period they will then go 'off privileges'. When 'off privileges', patients are confined to the off-privileges lounge with its associated behavioural restrictions. Restricted activities include sleeping in the chairs, watching television and engaging in pastimes (e.g., drawing). As far as possible, inappropriate behaviour is ignored ('timed-out-on-the-spot') and simply results in a failure to earn tokens. Aggressive episodes directed at another individual lead to time-out in the 'time-out room'.

'Time-out' is an abbreviation for 'time out from positive reinforcement'. This is an extinction procedure attempting to remove the individual from the opportunity of gaining positive reinforcement following aggressive behaviour. The patient is conveyed (voluntarily if possible) to a locked bare room where they are kept for a maximum of ten minutes and will fail to earn tokens for the hour period in which the time-out occurred. On very rare occasions intramuscular medication may be used to control the patient's aggressive behaviour. This only occurs when the patient's aggressive behaviour is not controllable within the system, or when it seriously endangers themselves or others.

Within the token economy a system of levels is in operation and is regarded as one of the primary methods of creating a therapeutic environment (Edwards and Roundtree, 1981). When admitted to the unit the individual is placed on Level One where the stringencies of the behavioural system are at their most severe. The weekly allowance of money is meagre and parole from the unit is allowed only with staff escort. Level Two, which can be earned by twenty-one days without a major infraction and with no more than three consecutive days off privileges, allows unescorted parole in the hospital grounds, a considerably more generous allowance of money and access to the hospital youth club. Remaining on this level for twenty-one days (again without major infractions or more than three consecutive days off privileges) entitles the individual to move to Level Three which is the highest level on the unit. On this level unescorted town parole is permitted, as are weekend leave and access to savings. Staff endeavour to ensure that patients find this level of privileges rewarding by the addition of movies, outings and a great deal of attention. Rules for remaining on Level Three are the same as for other levels and major infractions such as fire-setting and absconding result in a return to Level One, day one. The greater the number of times that an individual can pass through the level system, the greater is the opportunity for learning and a change in behaviour.

Assessment and Special Programmes

Ward rounds take place twice weekly when the patients' current progress and their treatment programmes are discussed. The ward round is designed to cover day-to-day management problems and to allow for a continuing fine tuning of the token system in order to keep pace with the changing needs of each patient. No matter how well a behavioural programme is designed, it needs to be adaptable to the patient's changing behaviours. A thorough assessment procedure takes place six weeks after admission and then at regular three-monthly intervals.

The OT, nursing staff, industrial therapist, remedial teacher and psychologist all prepare reports on the patient's capabilities and behaviour within their specialized areas. General behaviour and response to the token system are assessed via a review of the total token earnings during the previous three months by the number of meals lost, and by the number of time-out procedures required. A specially developed behavioural rating scale provides information on the patients' particular areas of difficulty and is completed independently by five qualified members of staff. This kind of behavioural checklist is used to complement traditional psychological and psychiatric evaluations (Edwards and Roundtree, 1981). Problem areas are ranked in order of importance and then become the patient's target behaviours which together make up the patient's programme. Examples of behaviours which might be targeted include biting or scratching others, shouting at others and manipulating others to get them into trouble. During the operation of a programme the patient may fail to earn tokens if they display the targeted behaviour. This is in addition to the normal criteria for token earning discussed previously. Alternatively the patient may be seen individually during a set period of the day, and special reinforcement which depends on conduct in the session is used. Programmes can be used to modify dress, hygiene, posture, overactivity and many other inappropriate behaviours. Burgess *et al.* (in press) have reported one such programme to address attending behaviour. The treatment sessions consisted of ward activities run by the OT. Token payments (separate from the normal token programme), which could later be cashed-in for edibles, were used to reinforce attending behaviour defined as head orientation towards the centre of appropriate group attention with eyes open and appropriately oriented. For the three patients reported the efficacy of the approach was demonstrated and was maintained after the programme ceased.

For particularly anti-social or resistant behavioural problems, a special time-out programme may be used; whenever the patient emits the targeted behaviour they are taken to the time-out room for two minutes.

Another technique on the unit is called 'over-correction'. Here, after the patient has performed a maladaptive behaviour they are made to correct the consequences of the behaviour and to do so long after its concrete results have been remedied. An example will make the operation of this method clear. A patient on the unit had a habit of overturning chairs if frustrated in any way. Whenever this happened staff members would overturn all the other chairs in the area. If the patient cooperates in the over-correction procedure they will earn tokens for the period. Many other types of behaviour can be treated in this way.

Problem Behaviours

Problem behaviours can be classed under a variety of different headings. For example, Edwards and Roundtree (1981) divided the problem behaviours in their population of adolescents as fighting, profanity, breaking and destroying property, stealing, running away and negative teasing. Here the target behaviours are described under the headings of manipulation, aggression and social skills deficits.

Manipulation. Although we may all engage in 'manipulation' to some extent, patients on the GHU do so to such a degree that it is a major problem for both themselves and others. Patients may lie, steal and deliberately try to cause fights between others. On the unit the patients' maladaptive behaviours frequently take the form of attempting to disrupt the system, for example, by threatening to report staff or attempting to play off one member of staff against another. These factors underline the importance of a 'tight' system with open lines of communication between all staff members.

Aggression. Aggressive outbursts, temper tantrums, threatening behaviour and physical attacks on others are all frequently seen. Patients may have a criminal record as a result of stealing, criminal damage, assault and arson as well as a range of minor offences. Patients also often display violence against themselves. These self-destructive activities can include suicide attempts or various forms of self-mutilation such as cutting or burning the arms, legs or scalp. Self-destructive behaviours are usually regarded as attention-seeking and are timed-out by ignoring the episode, taking only the necessary precautions to prevent more serious injury.

Social skills deficits. Most patients have some problems in the area of social skills. Swearing, verbal abuse, inappropriate touching and sexual behaviour such as masturbating in public are all problem areas. Self-induced vomiting, smearing of faces and hair pulling have also proved amenable to behavioural methods.

A large number of psychiatric conditions are associated with, and complicate, behavioural difficulties. All patients are carefully screened for organic disturbances which might lead to behavioural abnormalities. Parents are questioned as to possible birth complications and tests often reveal abnormal EEG results. A study of patients treated on the GHU has shown a relationship between abnormal EEG results (particularly focal abnormalities) and impulsive aggressive outbursts possibly leading to criminal behaviour (Bedford and Tennent, 1981). Where organic psychiatric disorder contributed to the behavioural disorder, appropriate pharmacological intervention may be helpful.

The Role of the Occupational Therapist

Assessment

As stated earlier, assessment is a very important part of the operation of the unit. In addition to the behavioural assessment procedure the OT conducts her own specialized assessments. Areas assessed include independent living skills such as cooking, shopping and self-care. Apart from these the OT assessment covers elements basic to performance such as attitude, motivation, mood, concentration, frustration level, comprehension and social behaviour. Assessments take place at three-month intervals and provide an opportunity for the therapist to note changes in behaviour as well as to designate specific aims for the next treatment period. Work assessments are conducted by the industrial therapy department.

Functional Skills

Many patients treated have deficits in the performance of functional skills. Where necessary, work may begin on self-care activities such as personal hygiene and dressing. Patients may need constant revision if they are not to lose even the most elementary skills. Domestic skills such as cooking and laundry are also requirements for independent living and may be included in both group and individual activities. There is a constant effort to keep the work on the GHU relevant to patients' needs and to their activities off the unit. It should be remembered, however, that although the OT is aimed to get the patients to reach their full potential in all life skills, this is often well below the level which would be required for independent living. The concrete aims for a particular patient will help determine which skills are concentrated upon. The examination of one activity will make apparent the way that practices on and off the unit are linked.

A vast number of skills are best practised in the community. These skills include a combination of functional, social and recreational skills. For example, on a typical shopping trip the individual needs to be able to cross the road, recognize social signs such as 'entrance' and 'exit', and know which shop to go to for a particular item. Within a supermarket the person must be able to find the item needed or be able to ask for it appropriately. Handling money and being able to make rough estimates of cost are also necessary if one is to plan shopping for the week or to buy more than one item. Many of these activities can be prepared for in a group setting on the unit. Patients can be instructed in how to cross the road and how to recognize social signs. Patients can also be introduced to meal planning in order to meet requirements of good nutrition.

Whenever possible, patients practise skills which they have developed during sessions by performing them around the hospital and in the community. Thus, on cooking periods not only do people plan their own meals but they also write a shopping list, estimate prices and, accompanied by a member of staff when necessary, go out and buy their own food. Many other activities can be included under the heading of functional skills. Patients need to be able to use public transport, tell the time, use the telephone, write letters and use a washing machine. The OT works closely with the remedial teacher in developing the more academic of these skills.

Patients are assessed and efforts are made to help all towards literacy and numeracy. Priority is, however, placed on work with younger patients. Courses are run in English, mathematics, child-care and homecraft. The remedial teacher is also closely involved in the teaching of functional skills where visual aids and practical sessions are used to educate.

Social Skills

Most of the patients admitted to the unit have some deficits in social/communication skills. Difficulties may have arisen for a variety of reasons. Some may stem from environmental factors such as poor parental modelling or early institutionalization. In other cases the difficulties may arise from specific complications of a psychiatric condition. In looking at social skills training on the GHU, one has to remember that the total ward prograrmme is geared towards assessing and improving individual social skills. This is done by prompting and applying token control throughout the whole day. In addition, there are more structured teaching sessions based on the model of Trower *et al.* (1978). Here approximately eight to ten patients work on specific areas in more depth. These sessions may include the use of role play for situational rehearsal, video and/or audio recordings for feedback purposes, and the imaginative use of 'props' to present a more realistic setting for such role plays. Every effort is made to help the patients generalize the skills which they have learned. Frequent activities are organized to provide realistic settings for patients to practise their skills.

Patients are given the opportunity to be responsible for organizing activities within the programme.

Recreation

Recreational activities are an important part of life on the ward and are organized by the OT. If being on privileges is not perceived as being highly rewarding, then patients will not work to attain it. Outings and visits are organized and provided without warning so that it is not possible for patients to manipulate the system by behaving appropriately only when it is in their interests to do so. Art work, roller-skating, pottery and bread making are all popular unit activities. Hobbies, team sports and games, and various leisure activities are encouraged to help patients structure their free time. These are, however, only available for those patients who are on privileges. Games and quizzes are enjoyed by most patients, and time is set aside for patients to plan and execute their own team pastimes. All of the more structured recreational activities are used by the OT to develop and reinforce appropriate peer interaction.

Work

Theoretically OT treatment is adapted to meet the needs of the patient. Assessment is carried out to isolate areas of deficit which are then practised until they are mastered and integrated into the individual's day-to-day activities. Industrial therapy (IT), by contrast, introduces an element of pressure and a requirement to conform to work standards which are shared with others (Wansborough, 1981). In practice the progression from OT to IT is gradual. Many of the activities run by the OT can be seen as work preparation. This not only means working on the social skills involved in job application and interviews, but also developing more basic work skills. In order to work, patients need to be able to concentrate, maintain activity at a certain rate, understand and follow simple verbal instructions, get themselves to and from work, and possess a sufficient level of manual dexterity. Work on all of these areas is begun in OT.

Patients are first introduced to IT on the ward, where they take part in short sessions using materials brought from the industrial therapy unit (ITU). Most frequently simple packing and assembly tasks are provided. As the next step from working on the ward, patients then spend short periods in the ITU itself, the length of time depending on the patients' progress and their other treatment needs. Full-time attendance at the ITU carries a number of benefits and is much sought after by patients. Firstly, there is the ideal of 'going to work'. Living and working in separate places are part of society's normal and approved model. Patients are aware of this and, like the rest of us, are at times happy to have a job. Most patients find the small assembly and packing work done in IT quite acceptable. Secondly, there is a greater degree of both independence and responsibility involved in attending the ITU. The ITU is a two-minute walk from the ward and patients could, if they chose, attempt to abscond while making their way to and from IT. Thirdly, since patients from all the behavioural units in the hospital attend ITU, there is an increased opportunity for meeting and socializing with new people. Fourthly, patients are paid and have certain other privileges such as use of a communal coffee lounge run by patients.

The behavioural system continues to operate during time spent in IT. Patients gain 'points' for acceptable work and general behaviour, and for GHU patients these are converted into tokens on their return to the unit after the IT session. A time-out room is located on the ITU for patients who become aggressive during IT.

Work in the ITU can be seen in two ways. Firstly, as treatment, IT offers a formal structure and a way of developing skills which may be later used in the community at large. Secondly, it can be seen in itself as an aid to independent living. Many patients will continue to attend ITUs or similar facilities after having made the transition to living with their family, in a hostel or in private accommodation. In many cases these options would not be available were it not for the continued support of an ITU.

Typically patients remain on the GHU for between one and two years. However, if at any time their progress has been sufficient they are considered for transfer to a pre-hostel ward within the hospital which offers a great deal more independence and personal responsibility than the GHU, but which still retains behavioural control by means of a system of points. Most patients resident on the pre-hostel ward work in IT or a sheltered workshop located nearby.

Effectiveness

Two studies have been carried out on the GHU employing the same basic research design (Fussey, 1983; Moyes *et al.*, 1985). To control for the effects of maturation a matched group was used. This was provided by comparing the treatment group — persons who had been treated on the GHU for a minimum period — with a group who had been accepted for a place on the unit but who for one reason or another were not admitted. A variety of rating scales were completed, mostly by the individual's social worker although in some cases the parents were also seen. A number of objective criteria such as living situation were also used. The treatment group was found to be significantly lower in ratings of aggression, odd behaviour and psychological disturbance. Perhaps more significantly the Moyes *et al.* study clearly shows the greater level of functional independence (as reflected in living situation) in the patients treated on the GHU one year after discharge. Although success in the sense of 'cure' is unlikely to be achieved, any improvement which results in minimizing the problem behaviours to a level manageable in some kind of community placement is a reasonable aim of treatment. This is especially true given the current view that adolescents who are sufficiently disturbed to require care in an institutional setting are one of the most difficult groups to treat (Kazdin and Bootzin, 1972) . With these limited aims in mind it seems reasonable to conclude that the effects of treatment are beneficial on the patients' future level of functioning.

Acknowledgements

The authors wish to thank the staff of the Geoffrey Hawkins Unit, St Andrew's Hospital, Northampton, UK for much useful advice, and Dr P. Eames, Consultant, and Dr T.G. Tennent, Medical Director, for permission to report on the work of the unit.

References

BANDURA, A. (1969) *Principles of Behaviour Modification*, New York, Holt, Rinehart and Winston.

BEDFORD, A.P. and TENNENT, T.G. (1981) 'Behavioural training with disturbed adolescents', *The News (Association for Child Psychiatry)*, 7, 6–12.

BURCHARD, J.D. (1967) 'Systematic socialization: A programmed environment for the habilitation of antisocial retardates', *Psychological Record*, 4, 157–67.

BURGESS, P., MITCHELMORE, S. and GILES, G.M. (in press) 'Operational aspects of attention in atypical mental impairment: A behavioural procedure', *American Journal of Occupational Therapy*.

COHEN, H.L. (1968) 'Educational therapy: The design of learning improvements', in SHLIEN, J.M. (Ed), *Research in Psycotherapy, Vol 3*, Washington, D.C., American Psychological Association, pp. 21–53.

EDWARDS, D.W. and ROUNDTREE, G. (1981) 'Assessment of a behaviour modification program for modifying disruptive behaviour of emotionally disturbed adolescent males in a residential facility', *Corrective and Social Psychiatry and Journal of Behavioural Technology: Methods and Therapy*, 27, 171–80.

EDWARDS, R.B. (1982) *Psychiatry and Ethics*, New York, Prometheus.

FUSSEY, I. (1983) *Follow-up Assessment of an Adolescent Behaviour Modification Unit,* Unpublished MSc thesis, University of Warwick.

KAZDIN, A.E. and BOOTZIN, R.R. (1972) 'The token economy: An evaluation review', *Journal of Applied Behavioural Analysis,* 5, 343–72.

MOYES, T., TENNENT, T.G. and BEDFORD, A.P. (1985) 'Long-term follow-up of a behaviour modification programme for adolescents with acting-out and conduct disorders', *British Journal of Psychiatry,* 147, 300–5.

SHELDON, B. (1982) *Behaviour Modification,* London, Tavistock.

TROWER, P., BRYANT, B. and ARGYLE, M. (1978) *Social Skills and Mental Health,* London, Methuen.

WANSBOROUGH, S.N. (1981) 'The place of work in rehabilitation', in WING, J.K. and MORRIS, B. (Eds), *Handbook of Psychiatric Rehabilitation Practice, Oxford University Press.*

Chapter 9

Occupational Therapy in Group Treatment

Mary Ann Bruce

Group approaches have been used in OT since the beginning of the profession. The multiple types of groups, their extensive use and the principles of group treatment have evolved over time and are evidenced in a recent survey of current practice (Duncombe and Howe, 1985), in the history of group treatment (Howe and Schwartzburg, 1986) and in the critically-reviewed professional literature.

Occupational Therapy Group Literature

The influence of each of the eras can be seen in the multiple theoretical principles applied in psychosocial OT today. These principles are in the OT literature and represent numerous types of groups. The four major types of theoretical groups identified are: (a) task-oriented groups (Fidler, 1984), (b) activity groups (Mosey, 1981), (c) developmental groups (Mosey, 1986), and (d) functional groups (Howe and Schwartzberg, 1986). Each is briefly described here.

Task-oriented groups. In 1963 Fidler gave an overview of the roles and functions of the OT in group treatment. Fidler proposed that the activity group was a laboratory for learning and that during activities interpersonal, intrapsychic and environmental forces influence the affect, learning and behaviour of patients. Therefore, to minimize stress, remediate problems, increase learning, promote function in one's environment and prepare the patient for performing in daily life, the therapist should process activities using a 'here and now' approach. Fidler states that task accomplishment is not the purpose of the group but hopefully the means by which purpose is realized; the purpose being to view and explore the relationship between feeling, thinking and behaviour and their impact on others and on task accomplishment and productivity. The OT who endorses this group model applies group dynamic principles in activity groups to explore group cohesion, problem-solving, views of reality, cause and effect relationships, communication patterns and the relationship between roles of functions of the group.

Developmental groups. In the late 1960s Mosey developed the concept of developmental groups which was originally proposed by Wilbauker. Mosey (1970, 1973, 1981) identified the interaction subskills which are needed to perform in each of the five groups. The five groups discussed here are in sequential order.

In the *parallel* group two or more patients come together to share space and work on their own individual activity. During the group the OT gives each patient feedback regarding their performance during the group.

When patients come together to interact casually and to complete a short-term task, a *project* group exists. The therapist plans the activity and patients share material, tools and space, and cooperatively work until task completion.

The OT in an *egocentric-cooperative* group provides democratic leadership and helps the patient to decide upon a group activity which can be completed in one to two hours or one or two sessions. Within the group patients express their needs of others, experiment with group roles and give feedback to each other regarding the group and activity process. Stress management, time management and assertive groups exemplify this type of group.

The patient in the cooperative group shares thoughts, feelings, values and common interests, etc. and gains satisfaction from sharing. There is no specific end product nor expected outcome. Values clarification, music, art and poetry groups are examples of this group.

The patient in the *mature* group can put aside his own needs for the betterment of the group and accomplishment of the group's goal. Patients assume social-emotional and task roles in order to produce an end product, i.e., an adult group which makes toys to give to deprived children in the community.

Activity groups. Mosey (1973) also contributed to OT theory and practice and the concept of activity groups. Activity groups, used for assessment or to accomplish specific goals, are experiences in which the group members relate around a specific task. The group is a social microcosm which provides learning opportunities for patients in order that they might live more independently in their environment. In an activity group the OT uses her knowledge of group dynamics and activity analysis in order to facilitate understanding of the interactions in the group and the outcome of the activity experience. In 1981 Mosey presented a taxonomy of activity groups: (a) evaluation groups, (b) task-oriented groups, (c) developmental groups, (d) thematic groups, (e) topical groups, and (f) instrumental groups. Each group is briefly described here.

Using a specific frame of reference, the OT chooses a short-term activity during an *evaluation* group to observe the patient's interpersonal skills and responses to the activity.

The OT uses a *task-oriented* group to produce a specific end product or service. During the production the therapist helps patients learn about their skills, behaviour, feelings and thoughts with the purpose of helping patients make changes which will improve their performance in their environment.

In *developmental* groups the therapist uses stage specific activities to facilitate group interaction. The activities are graded to promote problem-solving and task completion, collaboratively, competitively or independently.

Thematic groups provide didactic, directive and supportive experiences to help the patient learn daily living, work and leisure skills for functioning in a protective environment.

There are two types of *topical* groups: anticipatory groups and concurrent groups. In *concurrent* groups the OT uses activities and discussion to help patients gain the knowledge, skills and attitudes necessary for their present life roles. *Anticipatory* groups help patients identify future roles and then develop the knowledge and skills needed for them.

Instrumental groups are used to maintain the patient's present function and to promote optimum health.

Functional groups. The most recent model of group treatment is proposed by Howe and Schwatzberg (1986). Functional groups use purposeful activities to help patients learn about their environment. During the group the patient can practise and learn skills to achieve mastery and to gain control of the environment. These groups are intended to help people function independently and to adapt in order to be successful in self-care, work and leisure pursuits. Successful performance in the group does *not* mandate a specific end product. Success comes from the learning process which occurs during active group participation. The therapist uses activities and group dynamic principles to focus on the here and now learning experiences, to empower the group, to facilitate the participation of individuals in the group, to build upon individual and group strengths, and to bring about change.

As is evident from the OT literature and survey of current practice, there is a smorgasbord of choice for planning OT groups. One can choose to design a group based upon a particular frame of reference or a specific group type or model. Regardless of the basis of choice there are common elements in each group: the environment, therapist, patient and activity. When these elements come together in any OT group there are also common factors that influence the group outcome: principles of group dynamics and the frame of references applied. The common elements and the process which occurs in each group and the possible outcomes of group treatment are described in this chapter. The chapter is intended as a guide for planning and implementing OT group treatment.

Occupational Therapy Group as an Open System

The OT group can be considered an open system, a system which has a historical foundation and specific group elements which could be called its component parts or input: the environment, the therapist, the patient/client and the activity. The interaction of these elements is understood through principles of group dynamics and application of OT frames of reference (called 'throughput'). Within a specific framework, group dynamic principles are the forces which shape the group's outcome (output). The output reflects the individuality of each group experience. It may change the patient's thoughts, feelings or behaviour as well as influence those of the therapist and the therapeutic approaches which she endorses. During the group experience patients and therapist interact in a hospital or community setting within a creative, skilled or interpersonal activity to promote change. Individual as well as group changes occur as a result of the group dynamic forces which play upon the environment, patient, therapist and activity. The change which occurs may be fed back into the system and thus becomes input for future groups.

Group Elements

The elements that exist when individuals come together for a group experience can be considered the *input* into the system: (a) the environment in which the group meets, (b) the therapist, (c) the patients, and (d) the OT activity.

The Environment

The type of group treatment needed as well as the ultimate group outcome are influenced by the setting (environment) in which the group occurs.

Occupational therapists work within inpatient, outpatient, acute, long-term and community programmes. In many of these settings OT is one of the components of the milieu. Therefore, the OT's contributions to group treatment should be compatible with and complement other treatment offerings. As the therapist plans compatible treatment, there are several broad guides which provide the boundaries for OT groups. The clinical setting, group purpose, leadership, group composition, confidentiality code, dynamic process and treatment outcome vary for inpatient and outpatient groups (Yalom, 1983).

Inpatient and Outpatient Groups

Outpatient groups. Groups meet once or twice per week usually for a one-to-three-year period. During this time there is little patient turnover and more opportunity for group cohesion to develop. The group usually has six to eight patients who are functioning outside the treatment environment and have chararcter or heterogeneous problems. There is usually one consistent leader and the patient composition is controlled. Thus patients may have similar ego functioning. The group exists to maintain symptom relief, promote character change, and modify long-standing maladaptive behaviour. The group can also help its members to cope with current life crises and to prepare for future problem-solving.

Inpatient groups. The inpatient group is characterized by frequent change: rapid patient turnover, multiple group leaders and multiple roles for members in the group. Patients are room-mates and neighbours in the therapeutic setting and thus see each other frequently outside the group meeting. Staff members are group leaders, and may dispense medications, determine ward privileges or lead other groups. These multiple roles and responsibilities affect the group members' images and expectations of staff and thus the interactions of the group and its outcome.

The Therapist

The second group element is the OT and group leader. The OT comes to the group with her own personal history/needs, values, attitudes, beliefs, life experiences, etc.). Although this personal history influences group interactions and responses, the therapist's needs and concerns should not be the primary focus of the group. The therapist can sensitively use her beliefs and experiences to benefit patients and the group outcome.

The therapist has a repertoire of professional knowledge, skills and expertise (general, as well as those unique to psychosocial practice) which influence the multiple roles and responsibilities which she assumes in the group, the patient's learning and the group outcome. Specifically the therapist has a resource of multiple frames of reference and experience in applying them in treatment. She understands activity analysis and uses specific criteria for activity selection. She understands group dynamics and uses them to effect a specific group outcome. She is sensitive to the complexity of interpersonal relations that occur in group treatment and monitors these interactions to promote patient growth.

More generally the therapist's role is that of a 'gatekeeper'; a role which assures the patient's physical safety, which conveys an attitude of acceptance, caring and understanding and which values change. In this role the therapist provides a supportive atmosphere which promotes acceptance and caring attitudes among patients, provides an opportunity for risks and facilitates patient interaction (Bruce and Borg, 1987).

The Patient

The third element in the system is the patient. Each patient in the group is a person with individual physical, cognitive and psychosocial characteristics. The age, sex and physical stature of patients influence group interaction. For example, group members who are physically large may seem threatening to some patients or to staff, those with disablements or disfigurement may be rejected by group members, those who are attractive may be seen as better participants, and multiple age representation may lead to polarities in group discussions (Tubbs, 1984).

The patient's cognitive abilities will be evident in group interactions through the vocabulary which the patient uses, the depth of interaction which they desire (superficial, emotional, intellectual, etc.), the level of personal control which they desire in daily life and their preferred style of problem-solving) one of omission, independent, resourceful, shared, etc.).

Psychologically each person possesses a personal history which has shaped their self-image, personality, motivation, and attitudes and value system. Thus patients come into the group with feelings of confidence, prejudices and goals. They also will have a history of success and/or failure in daily life and home, work and community settings. These life experiences determine the roles which they have assumed and those for which they need to prepare. Roles such as those of parent, spouse, worker, friend require knowledge, skills and attitudes which can be evaluated and learned during group treatment. Thus all of these characteristics influence the patient, group interactions as well as the therapeutic outcome of the group.

The Group

The group activity is the fourth element in the system. The activities used in OT group treatment may be creative, require skill performance, be based upon developmental principles, promote problem-solving, facilitate interpersonal relations, or be cognitive, leisure- or work-oriented. Regardless of the kind of activities used in the group, the activity is to be 'purposeful'. Purposeful activities have to be considered the hallmark of the literature as well as many synonyms.

In 1983 the American Occupational Therapy Association clarified the term 'purposeful activity' in a paper by Hinojosa *et al.*: '. . . an activity becomes "purposeful" when it has "unique" meaning for the patient; when it utilizes the patient's abilities; when it helps the patient fulfill his life roles; when it helps the patient achieve his personal goals; and when it increases the patient's feeling of competence in self-care, work, and leisure. Purposeful activities are tasks or experiences used . . . to assess, facilitate, restore, and maintain physical, emotional, and cognitive function . . .' (p. 32).

In group treatment activities go beyond the use of time and have specific identified goals. The OT uses activities for many reasons. Activity can provide boundaries for behaviour and interaction. Usually, when opening a group, the therapist states the activity and its purpose which orients patients to the treatment experience rather than leaving them to wonder what will occur during the next hour; wondering what to do or say, worrying if they sound stupid, or what the expectations of staff and patients are in the group.

Activities which involve role playing provide opportunities for patients to receive feedback regarding their skill performance in simulated life experiences. Patients may learn to speak up for their rights, when to express affection and how to give support, how to ask for a date, what is expected in a job interview and how to ask for help.

Communication activities are used in OT groups with the intent of facilitating patient interaction. During communication groups patients hear about their interpersonal style, their ability to express themselves, and to be understood in their ease of interaction in multiple environments. Activities can also be graded and structured to promote success and to develop habits of daily life. Through activities patients develop new interests and learn to control their environment.

Regardless of purpose of the activity during groups, patients learn for the present and can acquire the knowledge, skills and attitudes which begin to build the bridge to the community. What patients learn from the group and how they build that bridge are influenced by the OT frame of reference which structures the group and the principles of group dynamics that occur during the group. The frame of reference and group dynamics are the throughput of the open system and are discussed next.

Frames of Reference for Group Treatment

In the OT literature multiple frames of reference are applied in group treatment. Amongst those listed which represent mental health are: (a) object relations, (b) behavioural, (c) cognitive, (d) cognitive-behavioural, (e) development, and (f) occupational behaviour (Bruce and Borg, 1987). Each of these frameworks is reviewed briefly here. However, the reader is encouraged to review the original source from which these summaries are derived.

Object Relations

A group based upon object relations gives emphasis to the process of the activity and the end product is secondary. Thus the therapist helps each patient to gain a better understanding of his social and task behaviour and strives to help the patient expand the ways in which he relates interpersonally and approaches activities. The therapist observes the following: (a) the methods of activity choice (e.g., indecisive, creative, careless); (b) the skills which the patient demonstrates (e.g., following directions, use of tools, eye-hand coordination); (c) the attitudes of members towards each other (e.g., caring, aggressive, empathetic); (d) the satisfaction with the group outcome (e.g., sense of accomplishment, frustration, defeat); (e) the feelings expressed about the group (e.g., individual patient responses towards each other, the task, interactions); and (f) the communication system (e.g., the quality of interaction, factors which promote or limit participation). The therapist then discusses her observations with the patient within the boundaries of their understanding and intended therapeutic benefit to bring about change (Bruce and Borg, 1987).

Cognitive-Behavioural Frame of Reference

Although there are multiple treatment applications of cognitive-behavioural theory, the predominant approach identified with this theory is the psychoeducation group. This group is an instructional model which utilizes contemporary educational activities, e.g., short lectures, audiovisual materials, worksheets and handouts, simulated exercises and homework. The activities are graded learning experiences to develop new knowledge and skills to achieve mastery; mastery meaning that the patients accomplish their individual goals rather than the performance demands of the established norms. A group of six to ten patients may meet in a classroom setting. Multiple patient levels of function in the group allow the patients to help each other, give feedback and provide support for risk-taking. Patients are encouraged to learn from each other and to work together during problem-solving. Programmes which exemplify psychoeducational OT are the life skills groups described by Lillie and Armstrong (1982) and the SCORE: Solving Community Obstacles and Restoring Employment programmes designed by Kramer in 1984.

Developmental Framework

Specific theories identified within the developmental framework are represented by Allen (1985) cognitive theory, sensori-motor integrative theory (Ayers, 1972; King, 1976, Ross and Burdick, 1976; Ross, 1986), recapitulation of ontogenesis (Mosey, 1970, 1986), and developmental theory (Llorens, 1976). Most of the developmental theories in OT place emphasis on the early years through adolescence. Of the theories previously mentioned only those of Mosey and Ayers adhere to the stringent requirement of stage specific, sequential developmental principles. In addition to these developmental approaches, Bruce and Borg (1987) discuss operant concepts related to adult development and emphasize the use of life development intervention (LDI) strategies during the adult years.

Therapeutic Factors

Although the structure and purpose of a group may vary, the therapeutic factors are common to each group and influence the outcome of the group experience. All the factors develop over time and some are more evident than others in particular settings. As summarized from Yalom (1983), the eleven therapeutic factors are as follows.

Instillation of hope. Patients at various functional levels have renewed optimism as they hear similar problems and see others take risks and change.

Universality. Patients meet persons with similar problems and experiences and realize that they are not unique.

Imparting of information. Patients gain implicit or explicit information regarding the meaning and management of their symptoms and feedback about their interpersonal style.

Altruism. From group interactions the patients learn that they can contribute and thus increase their self-value and what they have to offer.

The corrective recapitulation of the primary family group. In the group patients can re-experience family conflicts and learn new responses rather than use the maladaptive patterns which may be established.

Development of socializing techniques. During the group patients have the opportunity to listen, express empathy, respond to others and learn general social skills.

Imitative behaviour. Patients learn from other patients in the group and from staff role modelling.

Catharsis. Patients can learn to express feelings effectively in the group.

Existential factors. In the group patients can work through concerns regarding death, freedom, isolation and meaninglessness, and their relationship to the anxiety and pathology which they are experiencing.

Cohesiveness. The patients develop a sense of 'belonging' to a group and feel valued by the membership.

Interpersonal learning. The group is a 'here and now' social microcosm in which patients behave similarly to the way they do in the everyday environment. Thus change in the group can change the patient's interpersonal style and success in the community.

As the OT leads groups she will observe the therapeutic factors and may bring these observations into the patient's awareness. She may also adapt her leadership style to meet the needs of the group.

The Group Leader

In the early literature there are three types of leadership identified: autocratic, democratic and *laissez-faire* (Knowles and Knowles, 1972). The *autocratic* leader assumes authority for planning, implementing and determining the outcome of the group. During the group the autocrat presents the activity, assigns tasks, and sets and controls the boundaries for group interaction to achieve a predetermined outcome. The *democratic* leader values the capabilities of group members and encourages them to share in setting group goals, determining group activities, assuming responsibility for the group tasks and process, and in determining problem-solving strategies. The *laissez-faire* leader is more an observer than leader. Patients are given full responsibility for planning, implementing and controlling the group experience.

More recently the *contingency* style of leadership is endorsed. The contingency theory is one in which the group leader is flexible enough to adapt their style to the group situation and its needs. Thus within one group or week to week the group leader may need to adjust the leader strategy and be autocratic, democratic or *laissez-faire.*

The criteria which the leader uses to determine leader style are: (a)the quality of group interaction and the response desired (output); (b) the time available and necessary to accomplish the task; (c) the capabilities and satisfaction of the group members; (d) the group attendance and cohesion; and (e) the dependence-independence of group members (Tubbs, 1984). Plus the effectiveness of group function, the group history and the expectations which the group members have of the treatment experience can influence the leadership required and the group outcome.

Group Development

Throughout the group's life span as well as during individual group experiences, one of the dynamic factors which the leader monitors is the group's development. Group development is the specific or sequential pattern of events over time (e.g. Fisher, 1974) as well as within each individual group meeting. The sequence of events known as group development may have three or four phases dependent upon the theory which is endorsed. Tuckman (1965) has identified four phases which may be applied to OT groups: forming, storming, norming, performing. When people come together they need time to get to know each other and to be oriented to the purpose of their meeting. In OT a group warm-up exercise can facilitate group formation. As people begin to interact, individual needs, interests and value differences emerge and conflict may exist. During this storming period the OT listens for themes and tries to get the group to acknowledge similarities and differences and to focus on common concerns to begin problem-solving. The therapist does not gloss over differences to achieve harmony but may use them to help the group see alternative solutions, develop new standards and assume various roles in the group. Out of the storming will come group norms and group cohesiveness which will help the members work together as a group. For example, when the group identifies the expectations for attendance and participation and the roles for confidentiality or other codes for social interaction, the norming period will have occurred. Once norms are established the group can focus on its task and reach maximum productivity to achieve group goals.

As each of these four phases occurs, the therapist may choose to bring-the development process to the attention of group members in order to recognize their growth or to promote learning. The therapist may acknowledge individual or group accomplishments and at some point brings closure to the group or assists patients to terminate from the group treatment programme. In addition to the growth and understanding gained by patients from an awareness of group development principles, patients learn from the communication process which occurs during OT groups.

Outcome of the Occupational Therapy Group

The OT literature documents group approaches with all age groups and in many speciality areas. As with some other OT approaches, the research validating the effectiveness of group treatment is limited. Some of the studies most recently published contrast the effectiveness of activity and verbal group experiences. The studies suggest that the participants in activity groups show marked improvement in interpersonal communication (DeCarlo and Mann, 1985), that there is a decrease in symptoms (Klyczek and Mann, 1986), and that there is no significant difference between the two types of groups, but more importantly that each group member's response to an activity can vary (Froehlich and Nelson, 1986).

Occupational therapy groups are designed to meet the needs of specific patients and settings, to reflect multiple frames of reference or are adapted to achieve specific goals. In general the literature suggests that groups are used to develop daily living, work and leisure skills, to increase knowledge, to facilitate problem-solving, to produce an end product, to increase self-awareness and promote personal growth, to provide opportunity for socialization and to maintain a link with the community. The citings summarized here were chosen because of their relationship with other chapter topics included in this text. The reader is encouraged to consult the sources which are listed in the references.

Psychoeducational Groups in Occupational Therapy

Educational groups are based upon principles of social learning and competency educational principles. The group of six to eight patients usually occurs in a non-medical environment and in a classroom setting. After brief lectures or demonstrations, patients/students learn from each other during discussions, role plays or homework assignments (Bruce and Borg, 1987). Group topics usually have educational modules. For example, the SCORE (Kramer, 1984) is an employment readiness programme which has fifteen modules that are used during a twenty-four-hour (eight weeks, three hours once per week) treatment programme. Modules help the patient to identify the advantages and disadvantages of work, assess work and leisure interests and skills, suggest methods for selecting a job, give guides for the employment application process and provide opportunity to practise for employment interviews. The objectives of the SCORE modules are to teach employment seeking skills, to help the patient establish a realistic career objective, to teach the patient to sell oneself, to develop communication skills, and to improve amenities relevant to job seeking.

Another example of an education approach is described by Lillie and Armstrong (1982). They used an education approach with psychotic, depressed and character disordered patients who were seriously disabled. The groups offered structured learning through didactic and experimental activities in the life skills programme. The design of the programme's assessment goals and learning activities was based upon Hewitt's hierarchy of education tasks. The life skills programme educated students (patients) to alternate lifestyles and problem-solving strategies.

Group Treatment for Patients with Physical and Psychosocial Problems. Patients with multiple problems which are an outcome of a physical disability are also treated in groups. Group treatment for persons with traumatic head injury and with Parkinsonism are just two examples from the recent literature.

Lundgren and Perchino (1986) designed groups using Mosey's developmental group theory in conjunction with principles of cognitive level function. The inpatient groups were for those who were mostly under the age of 30, who had a traumatic head injury and who had functional problems. Patients had physical, perceptual, cognitive, social, emotional and communication problems. Thus their ability to interpret and interact in their environment was limited. They received individual as well as group treatment. During groups they worked to improve their organizational, judgment and reasoning skills, to increase their awareness of socially acceptable behaviour and their ability to interact with others and to improve their self-image and decrease their egocentricity. These goals were accomplished through structured, graded activities. Activities included life- skills training (e.g., map reading, locating community resources, ordering food from a menu), memory practice through games and opportunities to reason and abstract through stories, word scrambles, games and role play (what to do in an emergency, analyzing dangerous situations, etc.).

Another example of effective group treatment for the person with a physical disability is reported by Gauthier *et al.* (1987), who worked with patients having idiopathic Parkinson's disease in a group rehabilitation programme. This programme, a total of twenty hours, met twice per week for five weeks. The groups were designed to maintain mobility, dexterity and daily living skills and to provide re-education regarding the disease process. Each session had time for socialization, functional activities and educational activities. Sample activities include rhythm, music, singing and dancing to increase postural stability, and games and crafts to maintain dexterity. Guest lectures, homework and literature on Parkinson's disease to educate the patient and to collect data for the patient's future references were also included. The outcome studies of the group indicate that the patients maintained their functional status during a one-year period. They had a greater sense of psychological well-being, were less egocentric and had improved communication skills. They demonstrated an increased understanding of Parkinson's disease which decreased their fears and helped them view their symptoms more realistically than prior to treatment.

Group approaches also benefit patients whose psychosocial problem becomes a physical problem as seen with patients who have an eating disorder. The multiple groups more frequently identified with OT and described include assertive communications, creative and craft, cooking, pre-vocational, women's issues, body movement, stress management and relaxation, and community transition groups. In each of these groups the environment is structured and supportive, and patients are encouraged to set realistic short-term goals (sometimes ones which can be achieved in a single session). Goals are intended to help the patient gain control of their eating behaviours and then life in general, and to develop a healthy lifestyle — one which has realistic expectations rather than the perfectionistic ones so typical of the population with eating disorders (Bailey, 1986; Roth, 1986; Giles and Allen, 1986).

The Group Experience for Patients Who Function at a Lower Level. Kaplan (1986) combines the theory and model of 'focus' group treatment described by Yalom (1983) with the model of human occupation and proposes the 'directive group' as a strategy for treating patients with minimal level of function in a short-term setting. Patients in the group function at a low level due to hallucinations, delusions, organicity, severe depression, hyperactivity and other chronically problematic behaviours. The group of six to twelve patients meets five times per week for about forty-five minutes in a supportive, structured, predictable atmosphere. The co-leaders use activities to stimulate patient participation, provide a common task for interaction, and to promote skill development and confidence.

Each group session has four parts: (a) orientation and introductions; (b) a ten-minute warm up; (c) specific activity; and (d) wrap-up and group closure. When patients have attended ten to fifteen sessions and achieved the group goals (attendance on time, activity participation, verbal interaction), the patients are awarded a graduation certificate to acknowledge their accomplishments.

Conclusions

In summary the OT group as an open system model provides a guide for planning and implementing contemporary OT groups. The open system is a framework which allows the therapist to consider the elements in the group, the process which transforms the group into a therapeutic experience, and the possible outcomes which promote health and change for group participants.

The outcomes which were summarized from the OT literature reflect the rich heritage of group theory and practice. This heritage is one in which therapists have scripted a multifaceted role of OT; a role which gives viable options for treating many persons throughout their life span, with various problems and in numerous settings. These options not only meet individual group member needs, but also are compatible with mental health treatment philosophy and efficacy which can cope with the economic needs of health care. It is knowledge of one's heritage, careful planning, adequate documentation and creative adaptation of theory to practice which will carry OT into the twenty-first century.

References

Allen, C. (1985) *Occupational Therapy for Psychiatric Diseases: Measurement and Management of Cognitive Disabilities,* Boston, Mass., Little, Brown and Co.

Ayers, A.J. (1972) *Sensory Integration and Learning Disorders,* Los Angeles, CA., Western Psychological Services.

Bailey, M.K. (1986) 'Occupational therapy for patients with eating disorders', *Occupational Therapy in Mental Health,* 6, 89–116.

BRUCE, M.A. and BORG, B. (1987) *Frames of References in Psychosocial Occupational Therapy,* Thorofare, N.J., Charles B. Slack.

DECARLO, J.J. and MANN, W.C. (1985) 'The effectiveness of verbal versus activity groups in improving self perceptions of interpersonal communication skills', *American Journal of Occupational Therapy,* 26, 316–25.

DUNCOMBE, L. and HOWE, M.C. (1985) 'Group work in occupational therapy: A survey of practice', *American Journal of Occupational Therapy,* 39, 165–70.

FIDLER, G. (1984) *Design of Rehabilitation Services in Psychiatric Hospital Settings,* Laural, Md., RAMSCO Publishing.

FISHER, B. (1974) *Small Group Decision Making: Communication and the Group Process,* New York, McGraw Hill.

FROEHLICH, J. and NELSON, D. (1986) 'Affective meanings of life review through activities and discussion', *American Journal of Occupational Therapy,* 40, 27–33.

GAUTHIER, L., SALZIEL, S. and GAUTHIER, S. (1987) 'The benefits of group occupational therapy for patients with Parkinson's disease', *American Journal of Occupational Therapy,* 41, 360–5.

GILES, G.M. and ALLEN, M.E. (1986) 'Occupational therapy in rehabilitation of patients with anorexia nervosa', *Occupational Therapy in Mental Health,* 6, 57–66.

HINOJOSA, J., SABARI, J. and ROSENFELD, M. (1983) 'Purpose activities', *American Journal of Occupational Therapy,* 37, 805–6.

HOWE, M.C. and SCHWARTZBURG, S. (1986) *Functional Approach to Group Work in Occupational Therapy,* Philadelphia, Pa., J.B. Lippincott.

KAPLAN, C. (1986) 'The directive group: Short-term treatment for psychiatric patients with minimal level of function', *American Journal of Occupational Therapy,* 40, 474–81.

KING, L. (1976) 'A sensory integrative approach to schizophrenia', *American Journal of Occupational Therapy,* 28, 529–36.

KLYCZEK, J. and MANN, W.C. (1986) 'Therapeutic modality comparison in day treatment', *American Journal of Occupational Therapy,* 40, 606–12.

KNOWLES, M. and KNOWLES, H. (1972) *Introduction to Group Dynamics,* New York, Association Press.

KRAMER, L.W. (1984) 'SCORE: Solving Community Obstacles and Restoring Employment', *Occupational Therapy in Mental Health,* 4, 21–6.

LILLIE, M. and ARMSTRONG, H. (1982) 'Contributions to the development of psychoeducational approaches to mental health service', *American Journal of Occupational Therapy,* 36, 438–43.

LLORENS, L.A. (1976) *Application of a Developmental Theory for Health and Rehabilitation,* Rockville, American Occupational Therapy Association.

LUNDGREN, C.C. and PERCHINO, E.L. (1986) 'Cognitive group: A treatment program for head injured adults', *American Journal of Occupational Therapy,* 40, 397–401.

MOSEY, A. (1970) *Three Frames of Reference in Mental Health,* Thorofare, N.J., Charles B. Slack.

MOSEY, A. (1973) *Activities Therapy,* New York, Raven Press.

MOSEY, A. (1981) *Occupational Therapy: Configuration of a Profession,* New York, Raven Press.

MOSEY, A. (1986) *Psychosocial Components of Occupational Therapy,* New York, Raven Press.

ROSS, M. (1986) *Group Process: Using Therapeutic Activities in Chronic Care,* Thorofare, N.J., Charles B. Slack.

ROSS, M. and BURDICK, D. (1976) *Sensory Integration,* Thorofare, N.J., Charles B. Slack.

ROTH, (1986) 'Treatment of hospitalized eating disorder patients' *Occupational Therapy in Mental Health,* 6, 67–87.

TUBBS, S.L. (1984) *A Systems Approach to Small Group Interaction,* 2nd ed., New York, Random House.

TUCKMAN, B. (1965) 'Development sequences in small groups', *Psychological Bulletin,* 63, 384–99.

YALOM, I. (1983) *Inpatient Group Psychotherapy,* New York, Basic Books.

Chapter 10

Relaxation Training in Occupational Therapy

Diana Keable

The responsibility for providing relaxation training in psychiatric units often falls to the OT. This is clearly appropriate since relaxation techniques involve the active participation of the patient in treatment. In general the single most significant factor which distinguishes the contribution of the OT from other mental health professionals is a primary concern with the provision of 'active' treatment regimes. In this sense the term 'active' can be taken to refer to action-based approaches in the treatment of psychiatric problems, in which the patient is encouraged, literally, to work on their problems. It is apparent that most psychiatric conditions adversely affect function in many areas of everyday living. This is particularly so in the case of anxiety, which can cause widespread disturbances in the emotional, physical, creative, social and occupational aspects of lifestyle. Occupational therapists recognize the pervasive effects of anxiety upon the individual, and their approach is in tune with the rationale and methodology of relaxation training and many related techniques.

Thus a distinct responsibility is placed firmly on the shoulders of the OT. She is confronted with four major challenges:

1 to be well informed about the different types of relaxation training, their theoretical structure and procedural composition;
2 to be able to apply an array of relaxation techniques competently and intelligently in order to meet the needs of different client groups;
3 to be aware of contra-indications;
4 to be aware of anxiety theory and symptomatology, particularly those aspects which relate to relaxation training.

There are no easy ways to meet these challenges. Many of the issues involved are complex and remain unresolved. For example, no conclusive evidence exists about the clear superiority of any one technique over another, despite abundant research (Keable, 1985). Although the more recently developed comprehensive approaches to general anxiety (e.g., 'anxiety management training' — AMT) have shown promising results, as yet there is little guidance available on their clinical application. There is little evidence to indicate whether different techniques should be applied to specific problems. However, those with discrete phobias may not require the general approach of anxiety management programmes. Similarly programmes based on exposure to specific anxiety provoking stimuli will be awkward to apply and often irrelevant for more generalized anxiety problems. Additionally some patients present with largely physical symptoms, possibly requiring a muscle relaxation based approach. Still others present with difficulties which are largely cognitive, requiring a treatment approach based on cognitive restructuring methods.

It might also be said that differential relaxation, or 'relaxation in action', should be the particular concern of the OT. Differential relaxation concerns the practical application of relaxation skills to various aspects of daily living. The need for differential application has been addressed through various approaches; e.g., Progressive Relaxation (Jacobson, 1964), Simple Relaxation (Mitchell, 1977), and the Alexander Technique (Gelb, 1981). Jacobson emphasized the need to discriminate between 'primary' and 'secondary' tension. The former is necessary for the individual to carry out the task; the latter refers to excess tension, ultimately damaging to health. Alexander, whose techniques have been used widely by musicians and those in the sporting and acting professions, has described the 'use' and 'misuse' of the body. Misuse of the body while performing a task or posture is held to be the result of learning superfluous tension habits from an early age. Thus the recognition of excess tension during activity is an integral part of relaxation training. Relaxation should progress from the more passive positions (e.g., supine) to standing, walking and performing tasks in busy environments (Marquis *et al.*, 1980).

Finally, the contra-indications relating to relaxation training is not necessarily an innocuous technique, although it may appear to be so because neither drugs nor psychoanalytical procedures are normally involved (Jacobson and Edinger, 1982). Caution should be exercised, particularly when choosing suitable techniques for use with those clients suffering from any form of psychosis.

Anxiety

The Syndrome of Anxiety

While anxiety is a normal human response to stress, it becomes pathological when it is provoked in the absence of reasonable threat or danger. This is the kind of maladaptive anxiety which the OT is involved in treating. Cases of pure 'anxiety neurosis' are atypical in clinical practice. Anxiety symptoms can complicate almost any psychiatric condition and may be the principal feature. The multi-symptomatic nature of anxiety has already been mentioned, and cognitive, behavioural or physiological features may predominate in any given individual. The diverse manifestations of anxiety include: (a) acute physiological arousal symptoms, e.g., trembling, breathlessness, sweating, palpitations; (b) psychosomatic disease associated with chronic anxiety, e.g., ulcer, asthma, heart disease; (c) addiction/dependence on drugs or alcohol; (d) panic attacks and hyperventilation; (e) phobias, e.g., agrophobia, social phobia, claustrophobia; (f) avoidance behaviour, thereby curtailing travel, work and social activities; (g) impaired social and sexual functioning; (h) illness behaviour; (i) overdependence on relatives and friends, and excessive strain on relationships; (j) functional cognitive impairment, e.g., memory, task performance, concentration, decision-making ability; (k) irrational and negative thinking; and (l) loss of confidence and self-esteem.

The etiology of anxiety disorders is not straightforward. Causal factors may encompass genetic predisposition, psychodynamic and developmental disturbances, and stressful life events. A plethora of theoretical frameworks have been proposed upon which to base an understanding of anxiety. These have included psychoanalytical, physiological, behavioural, cognitive, sociological and existential models, but it is not possible to discuss these theories within the confines of this chapter. While it is certainly valuable for the clinician to have an in-depth knowledge of theoretical models, in the case of anxiety, sound and comprehensive assessment of the individual client's problems is essential.

The Assessment of Anxiety Problems

The use of a standardized assessment tool is recommended for pre- and post-treatment evaluation. For example, the 'state-trait anxiety inventory' (Spielberger, 1983) is simple and rapid to administer in the clinical situation and has been widely used in research studies involving relaxation techniques. The OT should also consider developing a structured interview or assessment battery tailored to the particular needs of the client groups being treated (see, for example, the Forensic Questionnaire in Chapter 14). From the OT point of view a simple tool to gauge the effects of anxiety upon function in a variety of aspects of daily living is preferable, e.g., work and social activities, physiological, cognitive and behavioural function. Simple self-rating scales are usually ideal for this purpose.

The next section provides an introduction to the major relaxation training techniques. They will be presented in the format depicted within Table 10.1.

Table 10.1. An Overview of Relaxation Techniques.

1 Basic techniques	
a *Physiological*	(i) Progressive/contrast relaxation
	(ii) Biofeedback
	(iii) Simple relaxation
b *Meditative*	The relaxation response
c *Hypnotic*	Autogenic training
2 Combined techniques	
a Cue-controlled relaxation	
b Anxiety/stress management	

Basic Techniques: Physiological

Progressive Relaxation Training (Jacobson, 1938).

This technique could be dubbed the 'father' of modern relaxation training methods. It involves the development of advanced muscular skills aimed at recognizing and releasing very small amounts of tension. A lengthy training is necessary, and daily practice sessions for one to two hours are recommended. Different types of muscle work, e.g., eccentric and concentric movements, are practised over all muscle groups. Jacobson described a powerful feedback loop which links the skeletal muscles and the brain. He observed that if a subject's muscles were relaxed, the person reported subjective feelings of calm. The reverse case was equally true in anxious subjects in whom levels of muscle tension were invariably high. Thus he argued that if a subject could be trained to relax their skeletal muscles, subjective tension and anxiety would also diminish simultaneously.

Jacobson's 'progressive relaxation' has been widely confused with 'contrast relaxation'. The latter involves exaggerated tense-release exercises and is probably the most commonly used relaxation technique of all. Unfortunately, although this technique is quick and convenient for use in the clinical situation, it is a crude approach and probably less effective than progressive relaxation (Lehrer, 1982). Contrast relaxation was evolved from Jacobson's original method by Wolpe (1958) for use as a part of his 'systematic desensitization' technique for the treatment of specific phobias. This approach is well known. It is based on the behavioural conditional principle of reciprocal inhibition in which the relaxation component is used to de-condition the fear stimulus. A hierarchy of fear stimuli is worked out initially with the client. The client is then progressively exposed to each item on the hierarchy while in the relaxed state. More recently within the treatment of phobias, programmes of exposure are generally preferred and the relaxation component is usually dropped altogether.

Clinical applications. True progressive relaxation is almost certainly far too lengthy and complex a technique to be appropriate for use within most OT programmes. While it is an exceptionally thorough training, more immediate and flexible methods are usually preferable in this context. Contrast relaxation has been adapted very widely for this reason, although its effectiveness is in some doubt. However, contrast relaxation may be useful in the initial stages of an anxiety management programme to facilitate recognition of muscle tension and the feelings associated with it.

Biofeedback

A large number of authors have contributed to the body of knowledge relating to the use of biofeedback in relaxation training over the last twenty years. Miller (1969) was one of the first proponents. This technique makes use of apparatus which enables continuous biological information to be made available to the individual about their own internal processes. Such information may be communicated in a variety of immediate ways via bleeping sounds, flashing lights or meter readings. The equipment may be used to monitor various modalities associated with arousal levels, e.g., heart rate, skin conductance/resistance, brain wave activity, gut mobility, blood pressure, skin temperature and voluntary muscle tension.

It has been shown that learned control can be achieved over processes under automatic control as well as voluntary muscle activity. Biofeedback was thought to work by providing information about the internal activity which does not otherwise reach consciousness. Using this information, the individual is enabled to develop control over these processes through operant conditioning.

Credidio (1980) and Goldberg (1982) have argued that while an individual can learn to reduce arousal in the specific site or system selected for biofeedback, this arousal reduction does not necessarily generalize over the body as a whole.

Clinical applications. Hamilton (1983) has suggested ways in which biofeedback can be used in OT to treat a variety of problems that involve elements of anxiety. However, accurate and reliable equipment is costly and may be inconvenient for use within the group situation. It has also been argued that ultimately ordinary relaxation training is more effective in reducing arousal than biofeedback (Silver and Blanchard, 1978). In spite of these drawbacks, biofeedback can be a powerful teaching tool when used as part of an anxiety management programme. However, the sophistication of biofeedback should not beguile the clinician into believing that it is necessarily superior to more simple methods.

Simple (Physiological) Relaxation (Mitchell, 1977)

This technique provides a refreshing alternative to the more well established approaches to physiological relaxation. Designed by a physiotherapist, it involves precise movements of the agonist muscle groups only. It is the opposing antagonistic muscle groups which are responsible for moving the body into the typical postures associated with anxiety, e.g., elevated shoulders, frowning facial expression, crossed legs. According to the precept of reciprocal inhibition, when the agonist muscle group moves the body part into a new (relaxed) position, the antagonist group must relax to allow the movement to take place. Clearly, if one group moves, its opposer 'switches off' to accommodate the change of position.

The technique also comprises the following elements: (a) normal breathing movements, slow and low in the chest; (b) focus of attention upon the new positions of 'ease' produced by the agonist muscle movements; and (c) individual choice of cognitive activities, which may involve a sequence such as a poem or a prayer — unpleasant thoughts or worries being ignored.

Mitchell's technique does not involve tensing exercises since she does not accept that muscle tension is consciously perceived. She asserts that proprioceptors and skin pressure receptors have pathways reaching beyond the subcortex to the higher brain, unlike muscle tension receptors. Thus the activities of proprioceptors and skin pressure receptors are exploited in her technique to help her train the individual to recognize the relaxed position.

Clinical applications. Mitchell's relaxation technique is quick and simple to learn and teach in the clinical situation. It also lends itself readily to differential application in stressful situations. This is enhanced by the learning of 'key' positions or movements which can be used to induce generalized relaxation during activity. Dimmed lighting and soft-voiced instructions from the therapist are not required and the technique can be practised virtually anywhere that is sufficiently warm and comfortable. Three positions are described for training, and these are described later.

As a physiological approach to relaxation, Mitchell's technique appears promising but still requires to be subjected to properly controlled trials before its effectiveness can be confirmed. As with other physiological measures, the technique cannot be expected to deal adequately with the cognitive symptoms and emotional distress associated with anxiety disorders. However, this technique could be used fruitfully as part of an anxiety management training programme to tackle the physiological aspects of anxiety.

Basic Techniques: Meditative

The Relaxation Response (Benson, 1976)

Of the clinically standardized meditative techniques of relaxation, Benson's is the best known and most widely used. Benson evolved his technique from the study of a variety of ancient religious practices and modern scientific knowledge of stress. He noted that there were certain factors to such activities as prayer and meditation which produce what he called the 'relaxation response'. He consistently recorded reductions in physiological arousal (e.g., oxygen metabolism, heart rate, blood pressure and muscle tension) in trials with transcendental meditators. Based on these studies, he designed a simple technique with which he achieved similar results. The technique involves four main elements: (a) a quiet, comfortable environment in which to practise; (b) preliminary muscle relaxation in a comfortable position with closed eyes, focusing on the natural breathing rhythms; (c) a passive attitude to mental distractions or worries; and (d) a neutral mental or focal device to engage the attention, usually a word such as 'one'. Practice should be carried out twice daily for ten to twenty minutes.

Clinical applications. Benson's technique lends itself conveniently to the clinical situation and is easy to learn. Once learned, the technique can be applied to a variety of everyday situations (e.g., travelling on public transport) without attracting undue attention. However, clients with acute symptoms of anxiety, particularly those showing marked cognitive symptoms, are likely to find difficulty in adopting a passive attitude. In such cases clients are unable to concentrate on the focal device and find themselves besieged by their worries during relaxation practice. This is particularly so because the practice is client-controlled, even in the initial stages. In this, however, lies the advantage of avoiding client dependence on the therapist.

Basic Techniques: Hypnotic

Autogenic Training (Schultz and Luthe, 1969)

Although clinically standardized hypnotic induction methods are available, 'autogenic training' provides an alternative which can be used autonomously by the client. However, specialized training should be sought in order to practise the technique, and OTs are amongst those who have done so. This note of caution exists particularly because the technique, in its entirety, is essentially a psychoanalytical procedure. More advanced stages involve visualization, fantasy and suggestion, and ultimately focus upon emotional conflicts and trauma. The use of this technique with clients suffering from psychosis is inadvisable.

Basic autogenic training utilizes suggestive phrases in order to induce the relaxed state or trance. Examples are: 'I am at peace', 'My right arm is heavy', 'My right arm is warm', 'My pulse is calm and strong', 'My breath is calm and even', 'My forehead is pleasantly cool'. The heaviness and warmth exercises move from the right arm to the other limbs in turn. A few minutes are spent contemplating each phrase. Two fairly short practice sessions daily are recommended. A passive attitude towards anxious thoughts or worries is cultivated during practice. The client is encouraged to see these distractions as part of a positive process in which the mind is ridding itself of painful material.

Clinical applications. While this technique may be a powerful way of inducing relaxation in certain cases, it is not suitable for more disturbed clients. Additionally, specialized training is required which may make the technique less accessible for many therapists. Continuity of training is also advisable, for both client and therapist, in order to master the skills sufficiently and develop trust.

Similar techniques based on suggestion include visualization and guided fantasy. These do have a place in a comprehensive relaxation training programme, but care should be taken not to encourage dependence on the therapist through their use. Therapist-led guided fantasy is more suitable for experiential and drama-related activities than for relaxation training, in which the aim is to encourage clients to achieve autonomous control over their anxiety symptoms.

Combined Approaches to Relaxation

Cue-controlled Relaxation (Cautela, 1966)

This method involves two main elements: a muscle relaxation technique — usually contrast relaxation; and the use of a cue word to facilitate the relaxed response. Appropriate cue words are largely a matter of choice, although such words as 'calm', 'control', or 'peace' are often used. Cue-controlled relaxation is based on a behavioural conditioning rationale. The cue word is held to become a stimulus to relax and thus control anxiety. While in the relaxed state the cue word is conditioned by the client repeating the word silently to themselves while breathing out. Practice is self-directed over a period of four to five weeks. The client should practise twenty pairings of the cue word with exhalation daily. Thereafter the cue word should be used whenever anxiety symptoms are noticed, until relaxation ensues.

Clinical applications. Cue-controlled relaxation is a useful self-help method. It is convenient and simple to teach and learn in both group settings and individually. This technique may also be used as part of an anxiety management programme. The cognitive element may help to reinforce physiologically-based techniques for clients with marked cognitive anxiety. Cue-controlled relaxation may be easily applied in a variety of daily living situations. It also lends itself well for use as an emergency method of relaxation in highly stressful situations. However, the physical relaxation technique usually used in cue controlled relaxation may be comparatively ineffective. A fairly high level of skill in physical relaxation is required before the technique as a whole can be expected to be effective. Thus it may be advantageous to consider using the cue word approach with an alternative physiological method.

Anxiety/Stress Management

Anxiety management has become a general term delineating the new comprehensive approaches to anxiety problems. Several distinct techniques have been documented including 'anxiety management training' (Suinn and Richardson, 1971) and 'stress management/inoculation' or 'cognitive behaviour modification' (Meichenbaum, 1977). Such programmes combine several types of relaxation, cognitive restructuring elements and behavioural skills training. The following components might be included in a typical anxiety management course:

1 general education about the causes and effects of anxiety upon the mind, body and behaviour;
2 various relaxation methods, e.g., contrast relaxation, breathing exercises, emergency stress control, differential relaxation, meditative relaxation, visualization;
3 cognitive restructuring or rational emotive therapy (RET) approaches;
4 realistic goal setting;
5 problem-solving techniques;
6 social skills and assertiveness training.

The anxiety management model acknowledges that anxiety is a multi-dimensional problem and attempts to tackle symptoms on all levels, i.e., physiological, cognitive, social, occupational and behavioural. Emphasis is put on replacing negative coping responses with an array of positive strategies, or coping skills, with which to deal with stress. Thus personal control over symptoms is enhanced, which is in itself a powerful tool for overcoming anxiety (Hiroto, 1974; Anderson, 1977; Johnson and Sarason, 1978).

Clinical applications. Anxiety management programmes can be readily adapted by the therapist to a wide range of needs and abilities. Programmes are generally presented in a closed group setting in the form of an ongoing course of sessions. Owing to the large amount of educational material involved, the use of written handouts or tapes is advisable. This should help reinforce the information given in the sessions and guide practice of the coping skills. Sufficient time should be devoted to gaining mastery over the basic relaxation skills. Homework assignments are an essential part of anxiety management courses and monitoring sheets can be used to record progress and check that practice is actually been done. A feedback session in which home practice is discussed should be an integral part of each session.

Acknowledgement

This chapter is partly based on material from previous articles by the author published in *British Journal of Occupational Therapy*, 48, 4, pp. 99–102 and *British Journal of Occupational Therapy*, 48, 7, pp. 201–4.

References

ANDERSON, C.R. (1977) 'Locus of control, coping behaviours and job performance in a stress setting: A longitudinal study', *Journal of Applied Psychology*, 62, 446–51.

BENSON, H. (1976) *The Relaxation Response,* London, Collins.

CAUTELA, J. (1966) 'A behaviour therapy approach to pervasive anxiety', *Behaviour Research and Therapy,* 4, 99–111.

CREDIDIO, S.G. (1980) 'Stress management with a psychophysiological profile, biofeedback and relaxation training', *American Journal of Clinical Biofeedback,* 2, 130–6.

GELB, M. (1981) *Body Learning,* London, Aurum Press.

GOLDBER, R.J. (1982) 'Anxiety reduction by self-regulation: Theory, practice and evaluation', *Annals of Internal Medicine,* 96, 483–7.

HAMILTON, A.M. (1983) 'Electromyography: Potential use in occupational therapy', *British Journal of Occupational Therapy,* 146, 316–18.

HIROTO, D.S. (1974) 'Locus of control and learned helplessness', *Journal of Experimental Psychology,* 102, 187–93.

JACOBSON, E. (1938) *Progressive Relaxation,* 2nd ed., Chicago, University Press.

JACOBSON, E. (1964) *Anxiety and Tension Control,* Philadelphia, Pa., J.B. Lippincott.

JACOBSON, E. and EDINGER, J.D. (1982) 'Relaxation training', in *American Journal of Psychiatry,* 139, 952–3.

JOHNSON, J.H. and SARASON, I.G. (1978) 'Life stress, depression and anxiety: Internal-external control as a moderator variable', *Journal of Psychosomatic Research,* 22, 205-8.

KEABLE, D. (1985) 'Relaxation training techniques — a review. Part Two: How effective is relaxation training?' *British Journal of Occupational Therapy,* 148, 201–4.

LEHRER, P.M. (1982) 'How to relax and how not to relax: A re-evaluation of the work of Edmund Jacobsen', *Behaviour Research and Therapy,* 120, 417–28.

MARQUIS, J.N., FERGUSON, J.M. and BARR TAYLOR, C. (1980) 'Generalisation of relaxation skills', *Journal of Behaviour Therapy and Experimental Psychiatry,* 11, 955–9.

MEICHENBAUM, D. (1977) *Cognitive Behavioural Modification,* New York, Plenum Press.

MILLER, N.E. (1969) 'Learning of visceral and glandular responses' *Science,* 434–5.

MITCHELL, L. (1977) *Simple Relaxation,* New Jersey., John Murray.

SCHULTZ, J.M. and LUTHE, W. (1969) *Autogenic Therapy: Vol. 1 — Autogenic Methods,* New York, Grune and Stratton.

SILVER, B.V. and BLANCHARD, E.B. (1978) 'Biofeedback and relaxation training in the treatment of psychophysiological disorders: Or are the machines really necessary?' *Journal of Behavioural Medicine,* 1, 217–39.

SPIELBERGER, C.D. (1983) *Manual for the State-trait Anxiety Inventory (Form Y),* Los Angeles, CA., Consulting Psychologists Press.

SUINN, R.M. and RICHARDSON, F. (1971) 'Anxiety management training: A non-specific behaviour programme for anxiety control'. *Behaviour Therapy,* 2, 498–510.

WILSON, M. (1983) *Occupational Therapy in Long-Term Psychiatry,* Edinburgh, Churchill Livingstone.

WOLPE, J. (1958) *Psychotherapy by Reciprocal Inhibition,* Stanford, Calif., Stanford University Press.

Chapter 11

Social Skills Training

David J. Folts

Social skills, the ability to interact effectively with others in a social-community environment, has been ascribed by society as a critical factor of peer acceptance. Persons having psychiatric problems, be they acute or chronic, have deficits in social skills. As a result, psychiatric patients are not able to communicate effectively or relate to the normal public. Thus the patient is at a significant disadvantage in becoming and remaining integrated in the community. Table 11.1 presents a list and a brief description of those social skills required for acceptance by society.

How many social skills a psychiatric patient possesses will decide the patient's adjustment and success in social functioning. Long-term patients often lack the conversational skills (Skills 1–3) which are the basic building blocks in mastering higher-level skills. These fundamental social skills are hampered by the following.

Psychotic symptoms. These include delusions, hallucinations, agitation and accompanying behavoural difficulties. Although neuroleptic drugs are effective in reducing psychotic symptomatology, other symptoms such as anhedonia and social isolation remain largely unaffected.

Reinforcement of the sick role. Patients spending many years in a psychiatric institution develop modes of behaviour requiring little initiative and adult responsibility. Long-term patients become apathetic, isolated and less able to function independently in a community. This pattern of behaviour has been labelled the 'Social Breakdown Syndrome' (Paul, 1969).

Disuse. Social skills may atrophy as a result of indifference and lack of use. Sitting quietly and not interacting for long periods of time allow basic social skills to wither away.

Concrete cognitions. This type of thought process is characterized by rigidity not allowing the patient to use insight to solve problems. Furthermore, this

Table 11.1. Social Skills Needed for Society Acceptance.

1 *Initiating a conversation.* Speaking to another person about a specific topic.
2 *Continuing a conversation.* Beginning the main topic of discussion, expounding on it, and responding to the other person's points of discussion.
3 *Terminating a conversation.* Allowing the other person to know through verbal and non-verbal cues that he or she has been attended to and then ending the conversation appropriately.
4 *Making a request.* Describing to a person how they can fulfil a desire.
5 *Requesting assistance.* Asking another person for help in a specific situation.
6 *Following directions.* Completing instructions as informed to do so and requesting any additional clarification.
7 *Active listening.* Focusing on the speaker and responding to the speaker's message through verbal and non-verbal cues.
8 *Giving directions.* Clearly explaining in specific steps how a task should be completed.
9 *Giving compliments.* Telling another person that something which they did was liked.
10 *Empathic assertion.* Acknowledging an understanding of another person's feelings, beliefs or wants while clearly stating one's own position.
11 *Criticizing.* Objecting to another person's behaviour while offering a suggestion for change.
12 *Expressing anger.* Telling a person about a justifiable annoyance that he or she has caused without humilitating that person.
13 *Expressing feelings.* Being able to define an emotion that is being experienced and communicating that feeling to another person.
14 *Admitting a mistake.* Disclosing to a person that an error was made which affected that person.
15 *Accepting criticism.* Using a firm tone of voice and direct eye contact in explaining what will be done about the mistake.
16 *Reacting to another's anger.* Acknowledging that the other person's angry feelings have been heard and calming the person so that the issue can be discussed.
17 *Responding to non-verbal communication.* Being able to identify aspects of non-verbal communication which can help to interpret a person's feelings.
18 *Dealing with mixed messages.* Identification of contradictory and sometimes confusing messages which occur when a person states something but acts in the opposite manner.
19 *Bargaining.* Being able to compromise so that each person's needs are met.
20 *Assertiveness.* Standing up for one's feelings, thoughts and actions in a non-threatening fashion.
21 *Problem-solving.* Being able to define alternatives to solving a problem and then choosing the correct one.
22 *Decision-making.* Deciding on a specific course of action which will be in one's best interest.

thinking precludes putting oneself into another's place, being able to switch from one aspect of a task to another and abstracting or being able to go beyond present-oriented situations.

Rapid pace of setting. Because of the large number of tasks that are completed during the day, staff are often not able to converse with the patient at the patient's request. Therefore, social initiatives are not reinforced.

Few opportunities to practise social skills. When patients have questions for staff members not available, different staff members relay the patient's concern without allowing the patient to make a request. Patients not fitting the passive patient role may be viewed as potential disrupters of the milieu. Since much of the patient's hospitalization is participation in groups, those patients possessing few social skills will be more intimidated in a group setting.

Division of Social Skills Group

Because of the differences in social skills needs, patients may be dichotomized into chronic and short-term chronic populations.

Chronic population. The patient who has been hospitalized for many years, being non-interactive and socially isolated, is more likely to require basic social skills training. This includes non-verbal behaviours such as smiling and eye contact, paralinguistic behaviours such as volume and speech duration, and conversational skills such as asking questions and giving compliments. When primary social skills have been acquired, the patient will be prepared for higher-level skill training such as job interviewing skills.

Short-term chronic population. Those patients who have been functioning in the community and who will be discharged from the hospital in a short time will require skills which help them communicate more effectively with family, friends and fellow workers. This would include interpersonal skills such as dealing with a mixed message from a spouse, bargaining with a demanding boss, and at the highest level dealing with complex feelings and ideas.

A Theoretical Model for Promoting Social Skills: Occupational Behaviour

When treating psychiatric patients with social skills deficits, clinical and methodological concerns require a conceptual model that provides the organizing principles for treatment. Reed (1983) has identified the major concepts of the occupational behaviour model.

Intrinsic motivation. This stems from gratification of performing or completing an activity (Florey, 1971). Intrinsic motivation can be divided into a continuum of behaviours named 'pawn' and 'origin' (DeCharms, 1968). A pawn orientation includes: (a) feelings of being controlled by forces outside the person's control; (b) not assuming responsibiity for one's behaviour; (c) not being responsive to feedback in the environment (e.g., another person's non-verbal cues); (d) viewing oneself as having few choices, and (e) few risk-taking chances; (f) no belief in skills as being able to influence the environment; (g) little motivation to obtain skills; and (h) external orientation due to belief in fate as governing success and failure.

An origin orientation includes: (a) feelings of being in control of one's life; (b) taking responsibility for one's behaviour; (c) paying attention to feedback as a way of improving performance; (d) wide range of personal choices seen; (e) moderate amount of risk-taking; (f) belief in skill as being able to influence environment; (g) motivation to seek opportunities in the environment; and (h) internal orientation due to expectancy of success or failure being based on skill.

Table 11.2 displays how these behaviours lie on a continuum. No patient is either a pawn or an origin since specific circumstances influence these behaviours. In psychiatric settings an unhealthy dominance of pawn behaviour is often observed. To encourage origin behaviour, every opportunity is seized upon to teach patients how they can influence their social environment through the use of social skills. As patients begin to build social skills, then the origin orientation grows. When patients meet with even the smallest of successes, through social skill acquisition such as initiat-

Table 11.2. Intrinsic Motive (Pawn-Origin).

External Control (Pawn)	———— (a continuum)	Internal Control (Origin)
The taking of few risks, ignoring or distorting social feedback and not paying attention to opportunities in the social environment.		Seeking out appropriate opportunities in the social environment, paying attention to social feedback as a means of correcting performance and engaging in a moderate amount of risk taking.
Disbelief in social skills. Fate/chance governs success/failure in social exchanges.		Belief in social skills. Expectancy of success/failure. Based on belief in social skills.

ing a conversation with a fellow patient, then the likelihood that the patient will utilize that skill rises.

Competency motive. This is an attempt to contact and master the environment (Wolman, 1973). When interacting socially, the competency motive determines the patient's adjustment and success in social functioning. Since psychiatric patients often display hopeless and helpless behaviour, they have difficulty perceiving themselves as being able to influence people directly. This results in observations such as severed interpersonal communication, detachment and self-imposed social isolation. The competency motive can be strengthened by patients learning social skills, thereby enabling them to exert an influence on their social environment. The social skills group can be structured to provide mastery experiences that foster self-initiated and self-rewarding behaviour

Achievement motive. This is based on experience in problem-solving tasks and involves meeting performance standards for task completion. Linked to the development of achievement motivation is independence training. Independence training allows the patient to function more autonomously, thereby reducing the length of stay for the patient and decreasing likelihood of future admissions (Florey, 1969). Since chronic and short-term chronic patients are deficient in many of the social skills necessary for leading self-reliant lives in the community, independence training involves teaching patients how not to be passively compliant but rather to make requests and respond with initiative to others' behaviour through well defined performance requirements for each social skill learned.

Problem-solving. This is a process by which a patient discovers the correct sequence of alternatives leading to a goal (Chaplin, 1975). Before patients are able to solve problems involving social skills, they first must be able to label and identify the difficulty. Frequently problem areas arise as a result of a lack of social skills and concurrent lack of knowledge about these social skills. Patients learn by identifying problems through discussion and activities. Next patients define alternative responses to methods not found effective in resolving communication blocks. As patients learn new social skills, problem-solving ability is increased and the availability of alternate responses grows. Patients learn specific problem-solving skills with an emphasis on the patient changing his behaviour rather than attitudes.

Decision-making. This involves formulating a plan of action and following through with it (English and English, 1958). Problem-solving and decision-making are interrelated because patients must have adequate problem-solving skills in order to make sound decisions. Although patients learn and practise social skills in a hospital setting, patients must decide if they are willing to use these skills when they leave the hospital. Patients are encouraged to role play specific concerns involving communication difficulties and then to plan how they can translate that into actual performance in the patient's real life environment.

Social Skills Assessment

Evaluation is performed to determine those skills required by the patient in order to make a satisfactory return to the community. These will be social skills which the patient does not possess or does not use in social functioning. Since the use of social skills can be hampered for various reasons (e.g., adoption of patient role, unfamiliarity with setting and staff, psychotic symptomatology), assessments should be completed by a variety of staff having frequent contact with the patient. This includes therapists, physicians and nursing staff who have twenty-four-hour access to the patient. Those assessment tools used to assess social skills and intrinsic motivation include the following.

Non-Verbal Behaviour Checklist. Since research has documented the importance of non-verbal communication, and since chronic and short-term chronic patients have major problems in this area, Table 11.3 illustrates a checklist developed for use during the initial OT evaluation.

Behavioural charting. This assessment can be completed by any staff member who has regular contact with the patient. Behavioural charting measures the frequency of an observed behaviour and can be used to record social skills use. A record is made of how many times during each period the specific behaviour occurs. A baseline of behaviour is established by counting behaviours prior to treatment in the social skills group. Behavioural charting continues to be done during the patient participation in the social skills group, as well as after the group is completed. This is done to determine if the target behaviour has increased.

The IE Scale (Generalized Expectances for Internal versus External Control Scale). This scale (Rotter, 1966) measures intrinsic motivation or the degree to which one feels controlled by forces beyond one is control of one's destiny (origin orientation). The patient's score is based on the total number of external choices. There are twenty-nine questions with six filler questions which are not included in the score. Eight external choices is considered the

Table 11.3. Non-verbal Behaviour Checklist.

Behaviour	Yes	No	Comments
Maintained eye contact			
Indirect eye contact			
Shifting eyes			
Facial expression matched message			
Animated facial expression			
Grimacing			
Frowning			
Body language conveyed interest and openness			
Open stance			
Closed stance			
Clenched hands			
Tapping foot			
Sat at appropriate distance from interviewer			
Spoke firmly with inflection			
Spoke at even pace			
Spoke at appropriate volume			

norm. Those making more than eight external choices would be considered more pawn-oriented. Those making less than eight choices would be considered more origin-oriented.

Social skills checklists. These are used to identify whether a patient is using a skill and can be used in conjunction with behavioural charting. Using a social skills checklist, a staff member familiar with the patient can indicate how well the patient uses the various social skills described. A good example is the Structured Learning Therapy Checklist which assesses those skills which patients need for community survival (Goldstein *et al.*, 1976).

Treatment Planning and Implementation

The following are nine steps used in treatment planning and implementation for the chronic and the short-term chronic social skills group, adapted from Tigges and Marcil (1987).

Step 1. Assessment review. Through the use of the previously described assessments including the non-verbal behaviour checklist, behavioural charting and social skills checklist, those skills which would allow the patient to master the many demands of a social environment are identified.

Step 2. Establish intrinsic motivation. A patient is given a pawn-origin rating based on the results of the IE scale and through direct observation of that behaviour using behavioural charting. This will also provide a 'benchmark' for how much different forms of reinforcement of skill behaviour will be required. The more pawn-like orientation will require more reinforcement for social skills and concurrent practice of skills outside the group setting.

Step 3. Exploration with patient of social skills problems. Assessments will be ineffective if the psychiatric patient does not view the social skill as relevant to their needs. A fundamental concept of OT is the use of meaningful activity. Therefore, if the patient's and OT's perceptions of specific social skill needs are similar, the patient will be more motivated to learn those skills (Goldstein *et al.*, 1976). The purpose of the group must be explained to the patient and time allowed for answering the patient's questions.

Step 4. Review psychological/cognitive status. When examining these criteria, verbal ability, concentration/attention span and psychotic symptomatology should be reviewed. Concerning verbal ability, the patient must have at least minimal fluency in speaking and be able to interact in a group. The patient must also be able to understand verbal instructions. Concerning concentration and attention span, the patient needs to be able to attend for a minimum of fifteen minutes per group session. Concerning psychotic symptomatology, the patient must have minimal delusional systems and have no hallucinations.

Step 5. Review occupational behaviour assumptions. The OT should review intrinsic motivation, competency motive, achievement motive, decision-making and problem-solving, to ascertain whether the social skills group is meeting those needs.

Step 6. Develop and prioritize goals. The first priority is having the patient learn sufficient social skills to allow them to function indefinitely outside the psychiatric hospital setting. Goals should be graded according to the level of skill deficiency. For example, making a request is a less complex skill than responding to the feelings of others. Yet both involve expressing oneself. At least one short-term goal should be established which the patient can accomplish during the first group session. This can serve to stimulate motivation in future groups.

Step 7. Obtain staff and patient cooperation. Even though patients acquire social skills in the group setting, ongoing reinforcement of those skills is a necessity. In-service training sessions can be held to educate staff members on how they can help patients to practise outside group assignments. Family meetings can aid in enlisting the help of those who will come in frequent contact with the patient after discharge.

Step 8. Review goals and progress. Performance areas consist of: (a) competency in demonstrating role plays, (b) level of group participation, and (c) follow-up of out-of-group assignments. At this time a further review of the patient's psychological/cognitive status takes place to determine the effects which this may be having on performance level.

Step 9. Modify goals and methods. If the patient is not able to comprehend the material which is presented, nor take part in a discussion or role playing which allows transfer of learning to take place, the treatment goals require modification.

Social Skills Training Principles

The following is a leadership guide divided into three parts: title and introduction, discussion-activity, wrap-up. It includes treatment recommendations for a social skills group consisting of an adult population of either short- or long-term chronic patients.

Title and Introduction

Although no more than five minutes are spent examining the purpose of the group and the topic of discussion, this is where the attention of the patient is kindled. The explanation includes the following points.

1 Much of the information collected will be commonsense.
2 Each patient has social skill ability but could benefit from improving that skill level. Benefits include reducing the number of person conflicts and stress in the patient's life, thus allowing the patient to achieve closer relationships with people.
3 Communication is a skill and like other skills improves with practice.
4 A comparison is drawn to specific patient's recreational skills and skill improvement through practice.

The introduction also explains how the topic of discussion is relevant and meaningful to that group of patients. Comments are personalized to as many patients as possible. Each individual should feel that there are elements in the discussion topic that are valuable to them. If the initial description is unclear, then the patient's interest and motivation may be lost.

As part of the introduction, the following learning points are used:

1 a definition of passive/non-assertive, assertive and aggressive behaviour, and of what such behaviours communicate to another person;
2 a clear description of how non-assertive behaviour results in depressed feelings, hopelessness/helplessness, and reduced self-image;
3 assertive behaviour is not appropriate for all situations. A common example is to think of an instance when someone had become extremely angry at them. Patients are then asked for the angry person's response to assertiveness.

At this point the discussion topic is briefly introduced and the leader is ready to progress to the second part — discussion and activity. When making the transition between introduction and discussion, there should be a logical flow. If the transition is vague or confusing, again patients may lose interest.

Role Playing

The goal of role playing is to provide a realistic rehearsal of a social skill that can be used in real life. When role playing, the following points should be considered.

1 In the discussion-activity phase the OT should be listening for individual problems within social skills in order to determine who should be included in the role playing.
2 The group leader should decide who will be role playing with those patients needing to practise social skills. Since role plays move towards increasing complexity, initially one of the group leaders should play the opposite role. This allows for the role play to be kept simple and limited. As an alternative, reliable patients may be chosen to play the opposite role.
3 The group leader will ask the patient chosen to role play questions concerning the difficulties in using the skills.
4 The stage is set by creating an atmosphere akin to a real life setting. Props such as a telephone, chairs, desks and drinking glasses may be used to help simulate a real life situation.
5 The patient is given concrete step-by-step directions to follow in practising the skills. The patient is instructed to see the role play through to its completion and not to step out of the role to make comments or ask questions.
6 The remaining patients are asked to listen for specific events in the role play. On conclusion patients are asked to give positive and negative feedback.

7 If a patient has a major difficulty completing the role play, the group leader can stop the role play and reiterate the directions.

Anger Management

Table 11.4 presents an anger scale questionnaire which is used for a short-term chronic group to cover learning points relating to the topic of expressing and responding to anger. Patients are instructed to estimate the degree of anger which they feel for each situation and then to calculate their total score by adding together all the numbers. They are then asked to check their anger rating. As each patient completes the form, it becomes personalized. Thus the interest level of the patient is higher and group discussion is stimulated by asking individuals their scores and personal reactions to the scores. Earlier discussion points on expressing and responding to anger can be re-emphasized.

Role plays are graded according to the needs of the patient. To ensure a greater likelihood of success, role plays should initially consist of more mundane problems encountered in everyday living. For a female homemaker this might be making a request of her husband to pick up clothes off the floor. As previously mentioned in treatment planning and implementation, family members and friends of the patient are approached to prepare them how to respond to patients when they begin to use their new-found skills. The ideal situation would have family members participate in the groups. This is also true of staff members. If patients receive positive feedback for their newly acquired skills from staff members outside the group, they will feel more competent in attempting to use these skills.

After a role play, leadership feedback should not only focus on difficulties in exercising the skill but also include social reinforcement for practising the skill. For reinforcement to be most effective during a role play the following suggestions of Goldstein *et al.* (1976) should be followed: (a) give reinforcement at the first opportunity after the role play; (b) give reinforcement only after role plays that adhere to points of discussion; (c) alter content of reinforcement given; and (d) give reinforcement in an amount consistent with the role play.

Wrap-up

The summary portion of the group should last no longer than five minutes. As with earlier parts of the leadership outline, wrapping-up is done in a

Table 11.4. Anger Scale Questionnaire.

Score your level of anger using this scale

0 = Very little or no bother
1 = Somewhat irritated
2 = Moderately upset
3 = Quite angry
4 = Very angry

..... You are talking to a friend but they do not answer.
..... Someone keeps interrupting you when you are talking.
..... Your car breaks down leaving you twenty miles from the nearest gas station.
..... You have waited in line for forty-five minutes at the grocery store. After the person in front of you pays for their groceries, the cashier tells you that she is closed.
..... You are trying to sleep but your roommate wants to listen to the radio.
..... A washing machine destroys your clothes.
..... You have planned on going somewhere with somebody but thirty minutes before you are supposed to be there they tell you they cannot go.
..... Someone tells you that your feelings are not important.
..... Your television set breaks down in the middle of your favourite show.
..... Somebody makes a mistake and blames it on you.
..... Carrying four cups of coffee in the hospital cafeteria, someone bumps into you spilling hot coffee on you.
..... A small group of people make fun of you as you walk past them.
..... Someone does not do their work and you get stuck having to finish the work.
..... Someone lies to you about something important.

Your total score: ....

Anger Scale Scoring Guide

0–22	The amount of anger you feel is very low.
23–28	You are calmer than most people.
29–38	Your anger level is average.
39–43	Your anger happens more often than average.
44–60	You become extremely angry and probably have angry feelings a long time after the problem has gone.

clear and concise manner. During the summary the OT should: (a) summarize points of discussion and reiterate the relevance of improving social skills; (b) ask if there are any questions about the discussion topic; (c) give patients who role play homework assignments and ask if there are any questions about what is expected; and (d) end the group by telling the patients when they will next meet.

Conclusions

There exist literally thousands of former psychiatric patients living on city streets, in boarding houses, hotels, group homes and community residences. Many will return to the psychiatric hospital because of marked deficiencies in mastery skills.

Much of a traditional psychiatric setting still depends on the patient's verbal communication ability. These therapeutic methods rely on the patient's ability to abstract and sometimes understand complex ideas and verablizations. These are skills not possessed by most short- or long-term chronic patients. Through knowledge of activity analysis and activity grading, OTs can utilize techniques in a social skill group that emphasize concrete examples, rehearsal of behaviour, social reinforcement, and the basing of specific social skills taught on short- and long-term needs of the patient.

In a psychiatric facility the OT is in a position to teach specific social skills that are required to function in a community environment. This is done within a context of the patient's needs, values and lifestyle. Since it is clear that many psychiatric patients are deficient in social skills required for leading satisfying and productive lives, the OT's mission is to identify and treat the patient by teaching social skills in the most effective manner possible.

References

CHAPLIN, J. (1975) Dictionary of Psychology, New York, Dell.

DECHARMS, R. (1968) *Personal Causation,* New York, Academic Press.

ENGLISH, H. and ENGLISH, A. (1958). *A Comprehensive Dictionary of Psychological and Psychoanalytic Terms,* New York, McKay.

FLOREY, L. (1969) 'Intrinsic motivation: The dynamics of occupational therapy theory', *American Journal of Occupational Therapy,* 23, 319–22.

FLOREY, L. (1971) 'An approach to play and play development', *American Journal of Occupational Therapy,* 25, 272–5.

GOLDSTEIN, A., SPRAFKIN, R. and GERSHAW, N. (1976) *Skill Training for Community Living: Applied Structured Learning Therapy,* New York, Pergamon Press.

PAUL, G. (1969) 'Chronic mental patients: Current status — future directions', *Psychological Bulletin,* 71, 81–94.

REED, K. (1983) Models of Practice in Occupational Therapy, Baltimore, Md., Williams and Wilkins.

ROTTER, J. (1966) 'Generalized expectancies for internal versus external control of reinforcement', *Psychological Monographs,* 80, Whole No. 609.

TIGGES, K. and MARCIL, W. (1987) *Terminal and Life Threatening Illness: An Occupational Behaviour Perspective,* Thorofare, N.J., Charles B. Slack.

WOLMAN, B. (1973) *Dictionary of Behaviour Science,* New York, Van Nostrand Reinhold.

Chapter 12

Psychodrama and Drama Therapy Techniques

Judie Taylor and Linda Burton

Over recent years there has been an upsurge of interest in the use of creative arts in their broadest sense for therapeutic purposes. It is not our intention to discuss all of these but to focus on the use of drama and psychodrama in different settings. While some areas of drama may require specialist training, we maintain that OTs should be encouraged to use drama and psychodrama techniques as valuable tools in their work.

In this chapter we will discuss several examples of our use of drama with both patients and student groups, hoping to show not only its value but also certain underlying core principles which are central to both OT and drama. We feel vindicated in the use of a variety of techniques, and as Yablonsky (1981) states: 'In many cases, the combination of individual counselling or verbal group therapy in concert with psychodrama maximizes therapeutic results.' This chapter does not claim to be the definitive work on psychodrama and drama therapy but is a discussion of personal experiences in the use of these techniques.

Engelhardt (1977) has said that OT 'functions as a health care profession precisely because of its concern with physical and psychological well being through activity and function' (p. 672). Here we can see the parallels between occupational and drama therapy's view of human beings as creative and spontaneous, or 'open systems' in Kielhofner's view. By choosing both these ways of working, we are attempting to break away from a more reductionist medical model (or 'closed system') to an open system view of human beings.

Modes of Drama

The sessions/examples we have chosen to discuss cover the three modes of drama as outlined by Jennings (1986): the creative/expressive, the task centred, and psychotherapeutic/insight. The 'modes' of drama are not completely separate but highlight a different focus and are seen as complementary. They have, however, been suggested as a means of underpinning drama therapy with a theoretical framework.

The creative/expressive approach. While all drama may be seen as creative, the creative/expressive approach emphasizes this aspect more strongly, the aim being to develop imagination and creativity. As Jennings says: 'Through the imagination we are letting go of our logic and allowing ourselves to wonder how things were, or how they might be' (p. 196). She sees the focus 'on the therapeutic experiences of the drama rather than on the analysis and interpretation' (p. 197). The therapist's view of the client in this setting is as 'creator and explorer'.

The task centred approach. The second approach is task centred, where the emphasis is on the learning of readily identifiable skills. It is related to the 'drama of everyday life', i.e., how we are as social human beings. The emphasis is on role repertoire and role flexibility which is why role play is the most common technique used. In this approach again there is no emphasis on interpretation or on analysis. We are not, for example, interested in why a particular skill has not been learned but in how we might encourage that learning.

The psychotherapeutic/insight approach. Finally, in the psychotherapeutic or insight-oriented approach the focus is on unconscious and latent material that is preventing individuals from healthy emotional functioning. Problems are not just 'acted out' but integrated into the life of the psyche through reflection. Within this approach it would be easy to say that the emphasis is on interpretation and analysis, but it is important to stress that whatever interpretation and analysis are made, they are not imposed on the client so much as explored by the client. Therefore, as Jennings says, it is important in this approach 'to be able to bring into consciousness, material that is unconscious, to make known what is known' (p. 199).

Because of confusion about the difference between psychodrama and drama therapy it may be useful to clarify what psychodrama is and to define some psychodrama terminology. The reader may well say that psychodrama is the same as the insight-oriented or psychotherapeutic use of drama. However, it is *not* synonymous with these terms. Psychodrama is a specific form of drama therapy developed by Moreno in the 1920s and 1930s in the USA. Originally it evolved from analysis, but in Moreno's words he suggested to his clients: 'Don't tell me about it, show me.' Moreno is emphasizing the power of action as a therapeutic medium, unlike psychotherapy or 'talking therapy'. The action may enable the individual to 'see' and 'experience' things differently without the fear of punishment for his mistakes. Psychodrama can provide a person with the 'unique opportunity for externalizing their internal world onto the theatrical stage of life; and with the help of the group present at a session, emotional problems and conflicts can often be resolved' (Yablonsky, 1981, p. 4).

Examples

We will consider two examples of drama with a group of mentally handicapped people to highlight both the creative/expressive and task centred approaches.

Example of the Creative Expressive Mode

The main focus of this session was the canopy (coloured parachute), used not only for integration but also to develop creativity and use of imagination. The warm-up consisted of staff and residents holding the canopy, and raising and lowering it at different speeds. All group members were encouraged to run underneath, swop places, attract other group members' attention; the aims being to focus attention and increase/stimulate communication between the group members. As the group warms up, the facilitator asks: 'What can we do with the canopy?' Various suggestions come from the group: 'Wave it up and down', 'Lie underneath it.' Each suggestion is used in turn. Then the emphasis shifts from the practical to the more imaginative. 'What could the canopy be?' 'A foundation.' A group member scurries into the centre, poking his head through the hole in the middle and looks down at the 'water' rippling around him. 'A wigwam' is suggested. As the group is enthusiastic, this idea is developed into the main activity. The group starts to construct a wigwam. 'What could we use to support the wigwam?' The group finds foam blocks to build the central support. 'What sort of people would live in a wigwam?' 'Cowboys and Indians.' 'What noises do Indians make?' The group makes whooping noises. 'What do Indians do?' 'They hunt with bows and arrows and shoot and live in wigwams.' The group members move inside the wigwam. 'What would we do inside the wigwam?' 'We'd have a fire.' We mime the lighting of a fire. One group member suggests we smoke the pipe of peace. This is mimed and passed round to all group members. 'We tell stories.' An attempt is made to tell a story but this requires a lot of prompting from the facilitator. Finally it is suggested that we sing songs around the camp fire. One group member starts singing 'Oh My Darling Clementine'. Other members join in and move on to community singing of other songs.

It is teatime, the singing finishes, the group comes from underneath the wigwam and holds the edges again. There is a ceremonial folding of the canopy with each member involved.

Example of Task Centred Mode

In this session the emphasis was on the actual life experience and the potential use of drama to encourage learning of life skills. The group members had been away on their annual holiday and arrived at the department with their holiday photographs. This sparked off much discussion and reminiscence with the residents eager to relate their experiences. Moving to the activity area, the facilitator suggested that the group could show what the holiday was like. The warm-up consisted of focusing the group's attention on the sequence of events. 'How did you get there?' 'Bus'. 'What did you have to do before you got the bus?' 'I had to put my coat and hat on.' 'What did you do before that?' 'Put my clothes in a bag.' 'What sort of clothes? Did you fold them?' The group is encouraged to mime the folding and packing of clothes into a case. One group member asks to be the bus driver. The group then moves to the creation of a bus with chairs. The bus driver then positions himself at the front of the bus, hands miming the holding of the steering wheel. This proves unsatisfactory for him, so he scouts around the room until he finds a 'hoola-hoop' which fits the bill. 'Who did you sit next to? What happened in the journey?' The bus stops. The group members file off the bus for a toilet stop. Back into the bus. Someone remembers singing 'We're All Going on a Summer Holiday'. This and other songs are sung. The group arrives at the seaside. 'What happened when you arrived?' 'We went to find our beds.' 'Who shared the room with you?' The group unpacks their clothes and then a series of activities follow, the group enacting eating in the dining room, playing football on the beach, and dancing in the discos.

To close the group, it is the end of the day. We mime getting undressed, going to bed, and going to sleep. The facilitator suggests that the holiday is over. We are going back to the department and when we wake up we will go and make a cup of tea.

Analysis

Although these two sessions have different emphases, the reader may be struck by the similarities in the way of working. Both examples encouraged spontaneity and use of imagination in a setting which is otherwise extremely ordered and structured. Both sessions are action-based, breaking the task down into smaller parts in order to build them up again into a piece of creative drama. What is also apparent in both sessions is the involvement of the patient in the decision-making process. They take some responsibility for the session, choosing the direction of the drama. The facilitator or teacher must get a group over its initial passivity and into the drama. If members see their own ideas take shape, they will be more ready to participate. With use of the canopy the initial passivity of the group became transformed into movement, through focusing of attention, and stimulation of ideas into drama.

It becomes clear, therefore, that the role of the facilitator is not to dictate but to act as a filter for ideas, allowing their development while maintaining a watchful eye on the action, ensuring it is contained and remains within the working area. These patients have to return to the reality of their living environment — the ward.

There is a danger in assuming that such a group of residents, who have spent much of their lives in the limited environment of the institution, have little or no resources to draw on. As the reader can see, not only do they have life experience such as their holiday, but have absorbed material from such other sources as television and weekly film shows. None of us had experiences of the Wild West, yet we would imagine and recreate what it might have been like. Here the facilitator is building on the residents' strengths rather than emphasizing their deficits, and increasing their 'role repertoire'.

A major difference we would see is the use of 'real life' events as the basis of the drama in the second example. These could be developed to encourage learning of life skills, e.g., 'eating out'. However, we would not see this being developed to point out inappropriate behaviour in a judgmental way, but as Jennings (1986) says: 'Who is saying I am unskilled? And what is going to be done about it? Do I change or does society? Do I have a choice?' (p. 199). Our answer to this question is to explore possible alternatives and consequences of that behaviour to help prepare these people for 'required situations, as a kind of rehearsal for life' (Yablonsky, 1981, p. 527).

To highlight the use of some aspects of insight-oriented drama and psychodrama with groups, we will consider a training group for third year OT students at Derby School of Occupational Therapy, UK.

Example

The use of masks. With this group there had already been an introduction to the use of masks. In this session the group is asked both to make the mask and to create its character. It is important to acknowledge the power and the emotion that can be evoked in their use.

Warm-up. Students are instructed to construct two masks within half an hour, using card and templates to standardize them. The masks must be of two opposites, e.g., good/bad, young/old, and they must be wearable. They can then use any material such as paint and shredded coloured paper to construct, embellish and decorate their masks. When all masks are finished, they are laid out for the groups to see.

Main activity. The intention is to wear and assume the role of a mask which the group members select, the only stipulation being that it must not be their own. The facilitator asks the group to be aware of the feelings and process involved in the selection. Should the member not get their first choice, will they be prepared to ask for it or take second best? The group members then find a space to consider and create one character of their mask; e.g., how would the character move, sound, what would be its name, age, history. They then explore the wearing of the mask firstly in front of the mirror, thus experiencing how it feels and looks. Finally, 'becoming the character' of the mask, they move, make sounds and interact with the other 'characters'. The facilitator now introduces a scene such as a street party, funeral, any group gathering, allowing the 'characters' to interact. The group improvizes a scene which develops spontaneously until the facilitator draws to a close. The party is over.

Closure. Time is spent in the deroling and removal of the mask. Within the group sharing, feelings developed by the wearing and leaving of the mask are explored.

Analysis

This third example highlights in some ways the difficulty of trying to separate the approaches into neat compartments. On the surface this session could be seen as creative/expressive. However, it also operates on an insight-oriented level. The aims were not simply the creation of masks and a piece of drama, but awareness of self and how we interact. People may have emotions triggered by the warm-up or main activity or else bring them to the session. The focus is determined not only by what emotions are evoked in the session, but also by what emotions people bring to the session. In this particular example one group member had a sense of being angry on arrival at the group. She displayed this by grumbling about the task, complaining about not being good at art and 'rubbishing' the activity. She was not able to locate an angry mask when making her choice and so projected onto it by converting it into an angry 'stomping' role/character.

One of the masks constructed was of a cold, superior computer-like woman. The group member who assumed its role disclosed that she had located those feelings within herself. They had been 'introjected' or evoked by the wearing of the mask. In the microcosm of the group people may see reflections of the macrocosm (or world outside). In this particular group one member became angry about not getting her choice of mask, protesting 'I'm always like this. I always let someone get what they want. I always come second.' This was not a flash of insight as the person was already aware of this behaviour. She was, however, surprised at, and aware of, the strength of her emotions accompanying this behaviour for the first time. She began to realize that the group was not telepathic, and would not be aware of her needs unless she stated them clearly. This was important new information. At a later stage she asked for space within the group to explore possible ways of asking for what she wanted.

The use of masks and further development into roles and improvization can be seen as a use of symbols and metaphor. This enabled work to be done in areas that may have seemed too threatening to confront verbally or directly without the vehicle of the masks. As Jennings (1986) says, 'The way into the unconscious is through symbols and symbolic re-enactment of a situation. The use of symbols for unconscious projection is staying with the metaphor, although bringing it into consciousness' (p. 199). If we stay with the metaphor, exploring it rather than seeking to understand it, we do not arrive at a 'fullstop' but enable the participants to continue.

At no point was there any attempt to analyse or interpret work in this session. The group members interpret and internalize what the session has meant for them. Very often the need to interpret lies within the therapist and should be explored within *their* supervision. There is much debate about the role of facilitator. It is important to note that the facilitator did not participate in these sessions as this may have resulted in 'underdistancing' or over involvement and a 'working through' of the facilitator's own work. The role of the facilitator was to establish boundaries and assist in encouraging a safe working environment where the group members' role repertoire could be developed, characters could be built and there could be a finding of 'other selves'.

A Further Example

We have chosen to include this example not only because it shows psychodrama technique but also because it developed out of the masks session.

The focus has moved from the group to an individual protagonist: the person who has elected to work and who will enact current difficulties or past traumas with a cast chosen from the group. In saying this one must appreciate that the whole group may be involved to different degrees as auxiliary egos who take on important roles within the protagonist's piece of work. Yablonsky (1981) sees them as having a dual purpose, that of extensions of the director and the protagonist in the session. The auxilliary ego may be a facet of the protagonist, e.g., his sadness, or a representation of an important person such as his mother, or work through identification in the audience role.

Warm-up. The introduction of theatre games or exercises as a warm-up is a recent innovation to psychodrama. Moreno himself would very often begin his sessions by talking to the group, uncovering their feelings, conflicts and current issues. From this dialogue a protagonist would evolve. At the beginning of this session the group appeared to get its 'second wind' in that there was much discussion about the previous masks session, with one group member offering himself as protagonist. A contract was made to explore this person's feelings which had surfaced during the masks session.

Main activity. The protagonist was distressed, having no idea where to start. At this point the role of the director is to encourage the protagonist to talk at a feeling level (rather than struggling to understand what is happening) in order to explore possible directions. The director, incidentally, was seen by Moreno as having three functions: producer, therapist, and analyst. Yablonsky sees the director as needing constantly to diagnose the situation within the group and to create an environment in which the protagonist can work. The director cannot make the protagonist gain insight but rather acts as a catalyst.

The protagonist in this particular instance identified her feelings through colour, referring back to the blue of her mask, and the feeling of coldness and confusion. The confusion is a 'here and now' feeling and the director seeks clarification as to the colour of her confusion. 'Blue is coldness, red is anger, yellow is power', she replied. The protagonist is encouraged to select people to represent these colours which are then developed into a sculpt. The protagonist then takes on each of the roles of the colours, 'rolling in' the auxiliary egos, giving her perception of what they mean/are, what they would say, and what they are like. The auxiliary egos then assume the roles and the protagonist places herself in relation to them in the sculpt. At this point the protagonist becomes more distressed and effectively frozen and unable to move. She talks of a 'black hole of despair'. The director clarifies:'What is the black hole like? Is there a bottom? Can you see it?' The protagonist is unable to answer. She is distressed and stuck. At this point the director asks the protagonist if it would be helpful to introduce a double or auxiliary ego to support and help free her. The double is an auxiliary ego insofar as they attempt to become the protagonist. They are used to enlarge the situation in order to help the protagonist's performance. The primary concern of the double is to give much needed support to the protagonist and is invaluable when the protagonist appears frozen and unable to express the underlying emotion. The introduction of a double agreed, one is selected from the audience who assumes the body position of the protagonist, placing themselves slightly behind her. The double is encouraged to speak as the protagonist in that position. The protagonist is instructed to correct them when they are wrong but to echo the double's words when they mirror her feelings. The protagonist becomes clearer, shifting away from the black hole: 'No it's not a black hole. I'm at the edge of a cliff and at the bottom of the cliff there are rocks. If I fall, I'll get mashed on them and there is nobody to catch me.' The director then encourages the protagonist to 'scene set'; a table becomes the cliff and members of the group becomes the rocks.

At this point the protagonist expresses a fear of falling and not being caught and held, describing how she has been let down in the past. The director suggests that it may be helpful to explore being at the top of the cliff and goes with the protagonist onto the 'cliff' (table). The protagonist identifies the people that are at the bottom, describing her feelings being at the top. Metaphorically speaking, she describes how she has experienced being dashed against the rocks. The director suggests that the protagonist might try experiencing falling, being caught and held by the other group members. The protagonist agrees and the 'rocks' link arms, forming a human cradle. In her own time she falls and is caught by the group members. The director enquires if there is anything else that needs to be done and if this is a good time to leave this piece of work.

Closure. Other group members are asked to share their feeling and any point of identification with the protagonist, the role being to support rather than to offer advice or criticism.

Psychodrama Analysis

Perhaps this example is unusual in that there was no structured warm-up because the discussion centred on the masks session. It was noticeable during this discussion that one group member assumed the fetal position and remained silent throughout, with the exception of complaining of the cold and putting on her coat. It was significant that her mask and role had been entitled 'Mrs Cold'.

One of the difficulties in the role of director/facilitator/therapist is putting the focus onto someone and taking away their right to be silent, particularly when there is obvious distress. In this case the director decided to ask this group member how she was feeling and what was happening to her. At this point she broke into tears and for some time was unable to speak. It was important that space was given to those tears without pressure to explain or justify them. As the tears subsided, the director acknowledged the tears and asked if it was important to explore them. The answer was, 'Yes, but I don't know where to start.' Moreno felt that it was not important to know where to start but that one does start. In effect, he saw potential for work and that being agreed, the role of the director was to facilitate a starting point. The director used material given, i.e., colours, cliffs and rocks, as clues to dictate the direction of the work. It was important that the protagonist set the scene herself, using everyday items as props to represent her symbols.

A recurrent theme throughout the psychodrama was not being cared for; metaphorically speaking, being smashed on the rocks. It is important to stress that this was the protagonist's perception of the outside world, and that psychodrama could not protect the protagonist from it. What it did accomplish was the new experience of being caught, held and cared for rather than being let down by people.

It is interesting to note that the director was aware that the protagonist suffered from asthma which was often precipitated by anxiety. Prior to working it was checked that she had her 'inhaler', but throughout her work and long periods of distress she had no difficulty in her breathing. Was this because she was expressing feelings rather than 'sitting on' them?

The three-dimensional sculpting of the colours, people they represented and their relationships gave access to new insights that endless discussion may not have achieved. The protagonist actually 'saw' those relationships and her role within them set out before her.

The audience had the opportunity to take part in the drama through the role of auxiliary egos and doubles, and also through identification. It became apparent in the disclosure of sharing that there was much identification with the protagonist, which helped support her.

Conclusions

It is important to emphasize the more equal and sharing atmosphere of the session due to the nature of disclosure about the past, families, feelings and fears. Over recent months there has been much sharing of particular fears about the closure of the hospital and moves into the community. Although we have not worked in an insight or psychotherapeutic way with this group we would see this as a possible future development. It is not only 'intelligent' people who have feelings and need to have them acknowledged.

In the training sessions involving drama therapy there is frequent formal course evaluation. Early in training students may want to learn how to do things 'to patients' and often see little value in exploring themselves. This, coupled with the compulsory nature of these early courses, results in a lower evaluation of the course. However, following clinical experience, in courses which occur later in training and are optional (as in psychodrama and masks sessions) there appears to be a change of attitude. Where the student has become more aware of the purpose of experiential work and recognizes the need to learn about themselves before helping patients to do so, the course is rated more favourably.

Is there a place for the OT in using drama as preventative rather than curative? As OTs move out into the community and are assigned to health centres and Social Services, is there a role for drama? We feel that we have shown the use of drama with the 'normal person' i.e., the OT student, and that our work does not have to be confined to those labelled 'sad', 'mad' or 'stupid'. In the present fast moving times is there a role for drama in prevention of feelings of alienation and stress? We would hope to see the OT working in the community in such specialist areas as with the terminally ill, the bereaved, the carers, with fostering agencies and self-help groups.

We recognize that we are not drama therapists or psychodramatists and may be lacking in drama training and experience. However, this should not deter the OT who has an interest in working in this area from exploring the use of drama and developing skills. Important considerations are the need for supervision and evaluation.

One of the possible problems as we see it is the pressure of quality assurance. In all the examples given the minimum working time has been three months, the maximum two years. In times of financial restraint we need to be able to justify the value of working in this way. It would appear that we are disadvantaged when the use of drugs can achieve a reduction in symptoms and not the cause. If ever we are to get onto the cause we have to accept that this will take time and perhaps the use of other techniques.

Landy (1986) poses the question in relation to the use of drama therapy: 'Is there a place for drama therapy at a time in Western civilization marked by a return to fundamentalist religions, an obsession with computer-generated information, even in relation to therapy, a compulsive stockpiling of nuclear weapons, and a faith in psychotropic medication to combat mental illness?' (p. 5). How can we compete against strong medication and the extensive use of computers? Is it not time to turn full circle to the original ideas of those OTs at the beginning of the twentieth century who presented a method which was both holistic and sophisticated in its approach to patients and similar to drama in that it saw action as its core?

References

ENGELHARDT, T.H. (1977) 'Defining occupational therapy: The meaning of therapy and the virtues of occupation', *American Journal of Occupational Therapy*, 31, 672–6.

JENNINGS, S. (1986) *Creative Drama in Groupwork,* New York, Winslow Press.

LANDY, R. (1986) *Dramatherapy: Concept and Practice, New York, Charles Springer.*

YABLONSKY, L. (1981) *Psychodrama,* New York, Gardner Press.

Chapter 13

Head Injury Rehabilitation

Gordon M. Giles

The OT has a central place in the rehabilitation of the severely brain injured. Recovery in this population can be seen as falling into three fairly distinct stages. In the first stage medical intervention is central in treatment and is directed towards minimizing the effects of damage already incurred (primary brain damage), preventing further damage resulting from the body's reaction to injury (secondary brain damage), and in managing associated injuries. In the second stage the patient will be conscious and medically stable and will most frequently be treated in a rehabilitation unit. The work of the OT focuses on the maximization of the rapid recovery occurring at this stage. In the third stage of recovery (which may last for the rest of the individual's life), the OT works to help the patient adapt to deficits. The major mode of intervention here is training. Residual impairments may be very significant.

The First Stage of Recovery

At this stage the patient has a reduced level of responsiveness (coma) and the OT's primary role is to help in the management of tonal abnormalities, prevent skin breakdown and to liaise with the family. Some therapists attempt to stimulate patients in an effort to produce an increased level of responsiveness. Although various forms of stimulation may increase arousal (as measured by heart rate, for example), the efficacy of stimulation in increasing responsiveness has not yet been demonstrated.

In the majority of cases at some point the patient will emerge from coma, will become medically stable and will be transferred from the acute trauma centre or neurosurgery unit where they have been treated to an orthopedic, neurological or rehabilitation unit where they will be seen more frequently by the OT. Medical problems frequently continue, however, and some of these may not have been recognized in the acute stage (Kalisky *et al.*, 1985). The OT should be aware of the areas where medical intervention may be helpful.

Neuropsychiatric and Neuropsychological Consequences in the Second Stage of Recovery

Neuropsychiatric

Typically as the patient emerges from coma there is a period of delirium which may include agitated and aggressive behaviour. If the patient speaks, the content may be incoherent and rambling, displaying disorientation for time, place and person. As the individual recovers (and depending on the severity of the injury), the delirium resolves, giving place to a condition still marked by memory disturbance and which may include euphoria with signs of disinhibition such as overtly sexual talk or behaviour which is out of keeping with the situation. The patient may be confused, irritable, tire easily and have difficulty in communicating their needs to others. Patients may appear as if in a dream state, and delusions and apparent hallucinations have been reported.

Memory. Any injury which causes a period of unconsciousness leads to memory disturbances, although in mild injuries the duration of the memory disturbance may be little longer than the period of the disturbance of consciousness. The term 'retrograde amnesia' refers to a loss of memory for events prior to the injury. The period of loss does not appear to be directly related to the severity of the injury and can vary in duration from a few hours or days to years. In some cases individuals have lost recollection of a recent marriage or other major life changes. Anterograde amnesia refers to loss of ability to remember new information subsequent to the trauma. Post-traumatic amnesia (PTA) is a form of memory disturbance which is related to the severity of injury. For the period of the PTA the individual is unable to recall novel events for more than a few minutes at a time. The individual often remains disoriented in time, place and person during PTA. In most cases PTA resolves — sometimes suddenly, sometimes sporadically over a number of days — and the normal operation of memory resumes. The individual will, however, never be able to recall their experiences while in coma or PTA. In some cases memory function does not improve or improvement halts at a level which leaves the individual with continuing memory problems.

In working with patients with memory disorders it is important for the

OT to understand the distinction between short-term memory (STM) and long-term memory (LTM). It is generally accepted that STM is the ability to retain a small amount of information for a brief period of time. Normally seven discrete items (plus or minus two) can be retained for no longer than a minute or so. LTM accounts for all material that is remembered for longer than a few minutes and which is not being rehearsed. Psychologists have developed a range of formal tests to assess memory function and the OT should be familiar with these. On a practical basis the therapist can develop some informal tests which may reveal areas of deficit. These may include asking the patient where they are, telling a patient a name and address and then asking them to remember it after five minutes and one hour of unrelated activity. Other useful tests are to hide a desirable object in the room so that the patient can see you do so and then later asking the patient to find it. Asking the patient to follow a simple route may also yield important information regarding spatial as contrasted to purely verbal memory.

Neuropsychiatric and Neuropsychological Consequences in the Third Stage of Recovery

There are no clear signs which can be used to divide the second and third stages of recovery. However, continuing and regular assessment will demonstrate when the patient is no longer making the rapid improvement characteristic of the second stage of recovery. On neuropsychological testing the patient will cease to demonstrate major improvements although functional gains may continue to be made. At this stage gains in functional ability are likely to be the result of new learning, a process which continues in the brain injured (Miller, 1980). The OT needs to pay particular attention to the patient's difficulties in acquiring and making use of new information.

Neuropsychiatric

The patients' families, initially grateful simply for the fact that their head injured relative had survived, may begin to realize that the brain injured individual no longer behaves in the way they used to before their injury and may not even seem like 'the same person'. This realization may be difficult for both the patient and the family who may require extensive counselling and support.

Neuropsychological

Neuropsychological consequences at this stage of recovery represent static limitations to learning that must be considered when teaching the individual needed skills or when attempting to effect behavioural change. Memory and attentional disorders are central but it must also be noted how an individual attempts to plan a sequence of actions and how difficult it is for them to initiate activities. Although individuals with even very severe memory disorders can make use of training, other types of impairment may significantly interfere with learning. Specifically, extensive damage to the frontal lobes seems severely to hamper learning (Petrides, 1985).

Therapeutic Interventions

While interventions which attempt to remediate cognitive deficits directly (e.g., memory practice) are not of demonstrable efficacy, internal and external strategies which result in behavioural compensation may be effective (see Giles and Fussey, 1987, for a fuller discussion). Internal strategies can be thought of as rules for thinking or behaving which the individual follows in order to improve performance. For example, an individual with a right-sided field deficit may learn to turn their head round to the right, thereby using their intact visual field to compensate for the damaged one.

The most obvious example of the use of an external strategy is the use of a diary or map. When determining whether to encourage use of an internal or external strategy, the therapist should consider the amount of effort likely to be involved. The more complex a compensatory internal strategy is, the less likely it is to be used. Simple internal strategies are likely with practice to become habits requiring no, or little, conscious effort to execute. Complex elaboratory techniques such as visual imagery (Patten, 1972) are intrinsically effortful such that it is easier for the subject (particularly those with problems of initiation) simply to use an external aid. The use of internal and external strategies requires considerable cognitive processing space which may not be available to the severely brain injured. When this is the case, the therapist can engage in specific skills training to enable the subject to perform needed tasks. There is now considerable evidence indicating that even the severely memory impaired can make use of specific task training. Goldstein and co-workers (1985) taught three amnesic patients a variety of useful behaviours (e.g., walking to the institution's canteen); generalization between tasks was not demonstrated. Similarly Glisky *et al.* (1986) demonstrated that memory impaired patients could learn how to operate a computer and retain such knowledge. Our own group has reported the day-today treatment of patients using such techniques (Eames and Wood, 1985; Giles and Clark-Wilson, 1987).

Central to learning most things is practice. Individuals without memory disorder may learn such things from one event but skills require repetition for mastery to be attained. Let us take the example of learning a language. If a student wishes to learn French, they need to practise French. No amount of practising Russian is going to help the student learn French. It is important to practise what is to be learned and not something else. Secondly, it is important to break the language down into component elements (words and grammar) so that the student can understand what is to be learned. Equally important, the student must practise putting the components together so that French is spoken and not just French words. Lastly, the student must overcome any reluctance to speak the language in public and must be able to initiate and execute the skill acquired at appropriate times. Similarly, when training a brain injured individual in a skill, for example washing and dressing, it is important to practise the skill. After a method can be arrived at which will allow independence, the task can be broken down into small component steps which can be used as verbal prompts. The therapist can initially provide all prompts and gradually fade them out by, for example, introducing a time delay or by asking the subject what they are to do next. The complexity of the behaviours that the individual can produce in response to an individual prompt will dictate how frequently prompts need to be provided and how exact the prompt needs to be. In order to learn how to organize showering, the patients may be able to respond successfully to the single prompt 'Get dressed' or may need to have this activity broken down into component parts. Patients need then to practise the activities in order to reduce the effort required to initiate these activities.

For many patients to learn, material has to be understandable, frequently repeated and motivating. A behavioural approach provides a framework for this type of intervention. In the author's experience additional motivators (such as chocolate or other 'treats') may not be necessary if the individual is already well motivated towards the task, and providing the individual with feedback about their performance by, for example, the use of graphs and percentages is sufficient. However, where extinction of an undesirable behaviour is involved, reinforcement of the desired behaviour is essential if staff and patient are to retain a positive attitude towards the programme. If the individual has poor drive, is under-motivated or is motivated to unrealistic or inappropriate ends, then more tangible reinforcers may be required. The type of approach used will depend to some degree on why performance breaks down. For example, in washing and dressing an individual may fail because, given their new physical handicaps and their difficulty in planning, they are unable to produce a successful strategy for themselves. Alternatively the individual may be undermotivated or resistive but be physically and cognitively capable of performing the task. In the former case a skill-building approach may be more appropriate. In some cases, however, the two problems may overlap and the individual finds it so difficult to dress that it is unrewarding and therefore does not do it. Here the individual needs practice of appropriate methods so that the amount of effort required to perform the task decreases.

A range of behavioural interventions is available which can help the brain injured control their behaviour or learn new skills. These methods are described in Fussey and Giles (1987a). What follows are brief reports of treatment based on learning principles with the brain injured. It should be noted that realistic life settings are the most suitable locations for the treatments provided. The OT's orientation towards function is central to the quality of life for the patient as the individual's level of independence frequently dictates future living situations and hence quality of life.

Case Reports

Patient D.I.

Patient D.I. was knocked from his bicycle by a car in 1981. He was said to have been obeying commands when first admitted to the casualty department but deteriorated within a few hours. A craniotomy was performed to remove a large extradural hematoma. Prior to surgery both pupils were fixed and dilated and plantar responses were extensor. Duration of coma is unclear but was at least seven weeks. Seen almost four years post-injury, D.I. showed marked impairments in all aspects of memory other than for occurrences prior to injury, together with significantly slowed information processing and poor ability to attend. Both expressive and receptive language skills were grossly impaired. Among his other areas of difficulty D.I. had marked social skills deficits. D.I. would stroke and fondle those around him in a very inappropriate way. Repeated requests that he not do this, as well as orchestrated group pressure in sessions devoted to social skills, produced no diminution in the behaviour. A programme was therefore devised in which when a staff member saw the target behaviour they would interrupt the behaviour (physically if necessary) and say in an authoritative voice 'Don't touch!' This programme had only limited effectiveness and as time went on even with the programme still in effect the behaviour once again began to increase. A second programme was introduced in which whenever D.I. produced inappropriate touch the behaviour was interrupted and he was escorted to a locked, bare room (time-out room) for two minutes. This led to a further reduction in his inappropriate behaviour to a level which staff considered to be appropriate. A comparison of the two programmes is given in Figure 13.1.

Patient Y.R.

Y.R was 26 years old when he fell three storeys. The little information about the early course of his recovery revealed that a subdural hematoma was evacuated and he was in a coma for between one and two weeks. Seen nine months after injury, Y.R. had recovered sufficiently to be living semi-independently (with support from friends) and was taking a short train ride to come to the treatment facility. The patient's memory was moderately impaired and he also had a moderate nominal dysphasia. He was unable to

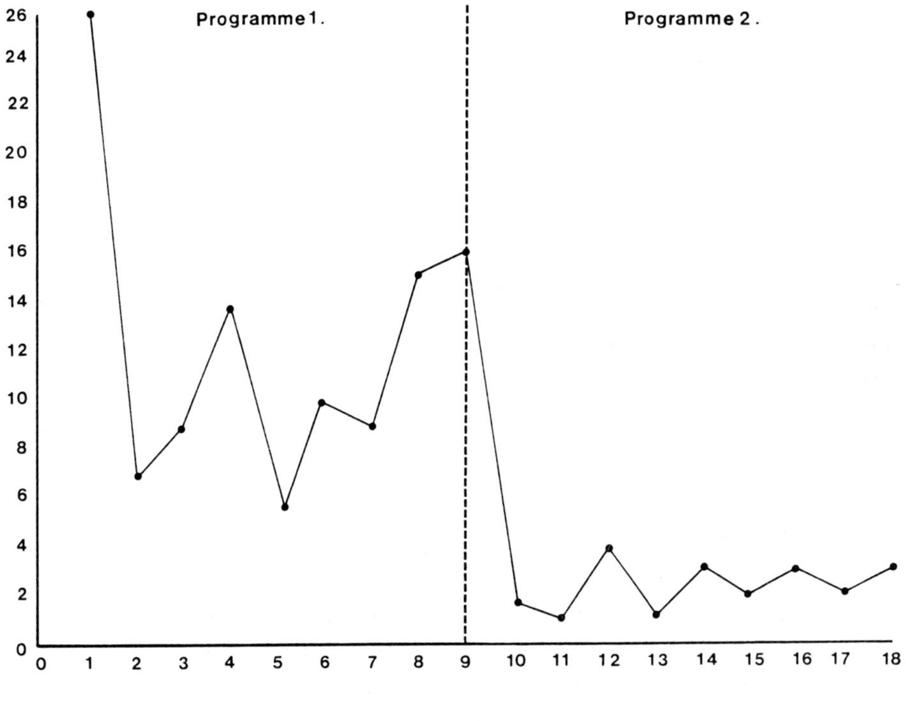

Figure 13.1. Response of Patient D.I. to Two Attempts to Reduce Level of Inappropriate Touching

name colours (but was not colour blind). While he was able to match colours which were identical on the dimensions of hue, reflectance and saturation, he was unable to state whether items varying on these dimensions were the same colour, i.e., shades of blue or different colours. Y.R. was unable to name or describe the use of food items. Y.R. when first seen reported eating in restaurants (which he could not afford) or living on milk or coffee as he could not cook for himself (prior to injury he had been a good cook). Although he could not distinguish food items from one another (he could usually distinguish food from non-food items), he was not otherwise agnosic. Work began on teaching him how to recognize and name fruits and vegetables and their uses. A limited number were used at first and others were gradually added. Y.R. practised with items in the kitchen and in the supermarket, and photographs were taken so that he could practise on his own. Figure 13.2 records his progress. It should be noted from the design of the study that Y.R. only learned food items that he was taught. At the same time Y.R. made himself lunch daily in one of the unit's kitchens and by discharge had developed a range of simple meals which he could shop for and cook himself. Concomitant work on the recognition and naming of colours also demonstrated considerable improvement using similar methods.

Patient D.F.

Patient D.F. (a 20-year-old male) was a baker for a large chain of grocery stores prior to his severe brain injury sustained in an automobile accident. Duration of coma was approximately four weeks which was followed by a period of delerium extending a further five weeks. When seen eight months post-injury, D.F. had severe abnormalities of tone affecting his left side, more pronounced in the lower than upper extremity. Heterotopic ossification in the left elbow limited extension by ten degrees. D.F.'s memory was significantly impaired; immediate recall of a short story was negligible and delayed recall was absent. D.F. required considerable assistance both physically and with prompts to be able to shower himself so a programme was designed to help him learn how to shower independently. The programme had two essential ingredients. The first of these involved devising a system by which D.F. could physically manage the task. The second involved breaking the task down into component steps which could be used as prompts and used to teach a routine to D.F. A programme was designed which incorporated the smallest number of prompts necessary for the patient to complete the task. Table 13.1 shows the individual prompts in D.F.'s showering programme and Figure 13.3 shows the number of prompts

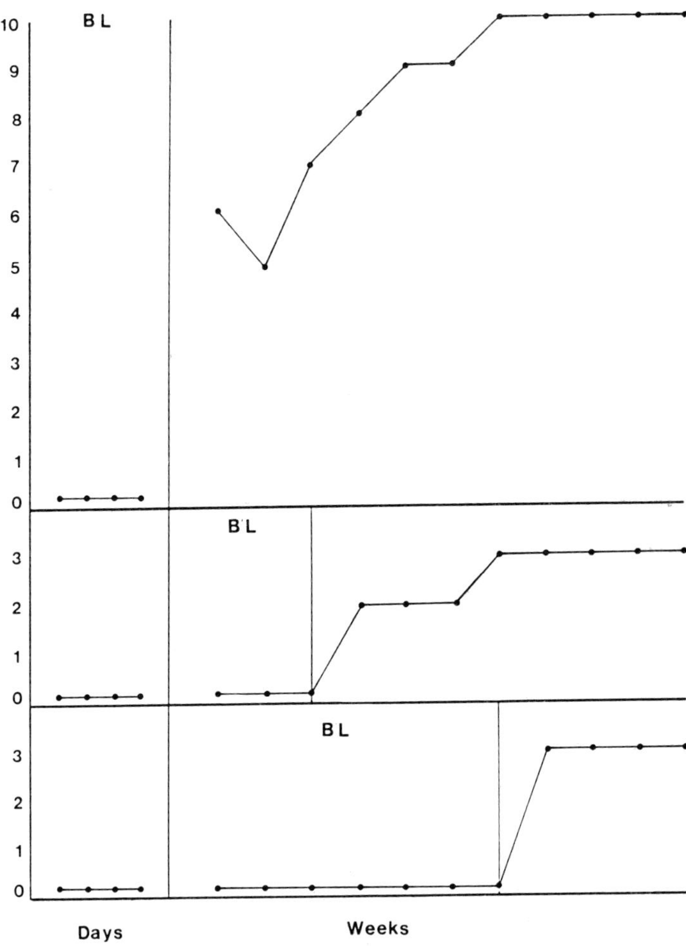

Figure 13.2. Multiple Baselines of Number of Fruits and Vegetables Correctly Named

required on each occasion until independence was achieved in the third treatment week.

Conclusions

This chapter has provided a brief overview of some of the issues involved in attempting to retrain the severely brain injured. The author's own experience would suggest that intervention may continue to be effective many years after injury. Individuals may have a limited ability to adapt

Table 13.1. Showering Programme for Patient D.F.

1	Get into wheelchair.
2	Take off pyjamas.
3	Put on shoes.
4	Put on bathrobe.
5	Collect towel and socks.
6	Go to the shower room.
7	Position wheelchair.
8	Transfer.
9	Take off shoes.
10	Shower.
11	Dry off.
12	Put on socks and shoes.
13	Put on bathrobe.
14	Transfer.
15	Go to room and get dressed.

spontaneously to environmental changes and may require repeated bouts of training as the circumstances alter. For example, a brain injured adult may have lived close to independency in the community with minimum support from an aged relative but when the relative dies the individual can no longer manage. Training in a new environment with a new set of supports may be all that is needed to re-establish independence. A small but growing number of single case reports (Giles and Clark-Wilson, 1987) and large group studies (Eames and Wood, 1985) attest to the impact of active and appropriate intervention in the third stage of recovery.

Unfortunately no single individual or body has responsibility for the continuing elevation of need and resource allocation for the brain injured. In few other areas is the need for such an integrated service so desperate (Fussey and Giles, 1987b). Frequently individuals are discharged home to the care of family without adequate follow-up services or support.

Issues which should be addressed in the management of this population include the individual's response to injury (psychosocial functioning), family issues, cognitive, behavioural and physical deficits, social skills, psychiatric disturbance and vocational work and residence issues. An integrated management service should include an acute trauma/neurosurgical unit, psychiatric and psychological consultation, an acute rehabilitation unit, an applied behavioural engineering unit, transitional living facilities, work, pre-vocational, and educational community programmes, a skilled nursing unit and community residential placements with varying levels of support. Other than where medical considerations are paramount, the OT role in managing and executing these services should be central.

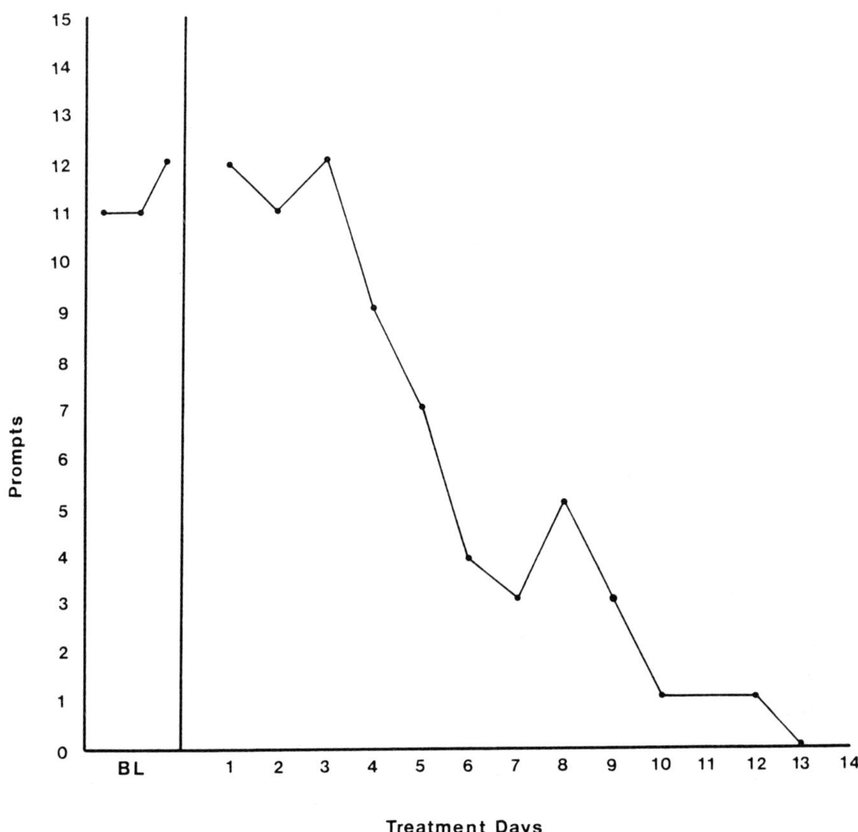

Figure 13.3. Number of Prompts Required by Patient D.F. to Carry Out Morning Showering Programme

Acknowledgments

The author wishes to thank Jeffrey Samuels, MD, Medical Director, Michael Shore, PhD, Director of Neuropsychological Services, and Leslie Paine, MOT, Program Director, all of Transitions: Bay Area Head Recovery Center, for commenting on an earlier draft of this chapter.

References

EAMES, P. and WOOD, R. (1985) 'Rehabilitation after severe brain injury: A follow-up study of a behaviour modification approach, *Journal of Neurology, Neurosurgery, and Psychiatry*, 48, 623–19.

FUSSEY, I. and GILES, G.M. (1987a) *Rehabilitation of the Severely Brain Injured Adult: A Practical Approach,* Croom Helm

FUSSEY, I. and GILES, G.M. (1987b) 'The future of brain injury rehabilitation', in FUSSEY, I. and GILES, G.M. (Eds), *Rehabilitation of the Severely Brain Injured Adult: A Practical Approach,* Croom Helm

GILES, G.M. and CLARK-WILSON, J. (1987) 'Functional skills training in severe brain injury', in FUSSEY, I. and GILES, G.M. (Eds), *Rehabilitation of the Severely Brain Injured Adult: A Practical Approach,* Croom Helm

GILES, G.M. and FUSSEY, I. (1987) 'Models of brain injury rehabilitation: From theory to practice', in FUSSEY, I. and GILES, G.M. (Eds), *Rehabilitation of the Severely Brain Injured Adult: A Practical Approach,* Croom Helm

GLISKY, E.L., SCHACTER, D.L. and TULVIN, E. (1986) 'Computer learning by memory-impaired patients: Acquisition and retention of complex knowledge', *Neuropsychologia,* 24, 313–28.

GOLDSTEIN, G., RYAN, C., TURNAR, S.M., KANAGY, M., BARRY, K. and KELLY, L. (1985) 'Three methods of memory training for severely ammnesic patients', *Behaviour Modification,* 9, 357–74.

KALISKY, Z., MORRISON, D.P., MEYER, C.A. and von LAUFEN, A. (1985) 'Medical problems encountered during rehabilitation of patients with head injury', *Archives of Physical Medicine and Rehabilitation,* 66, 25–9.

MILLER, E. (1980) 'The training characteristics of severely head injured patients: A preliminary study', *Journal of Neurology, Neurosurgery, and Psychiatry,* 43, 525–8.

PATTEN, B.M. (1972) 'The ancient art of memory: Usefulness in treatment', *Archives of Neurology,* 26, 25–31.

PETRIDES, M. (1985) 'Deficits on conditional and associative-learning tasks after frontal and temporal lobe lesions in man', *Neuropsychologia,* 23, 601–14.

SHIFFRIN, R.M. and SCHNEIDER, W. (1977) 'Controlled and automatic information processing: II. Perceptual learning, automatic attending, and a general theory', *Psychological Review,* 84, 127–90.

Chapter 14

Occupational Therapy in Forensic Psychiatry

Chris Lloyd

Forensic psychiatry, the intermix of psychiatry and the law, is not a new field but it is only over the last decade that the role of the OT has emerged (Smith, 1984). The OT working in a forensic psychiatric setting has had to face the unique challenge of developing specific assessment and treatment methods for a population of patients who have a history of aggression and formidable psychiatric and legal difficulties (Rice, 1985).

Programme Planning

Many changes have taken place in mental health care, including the emergence of a variety of new disciplines competing with OT to provide programmes based on normal activities with a practical orientation. This has resulted in increasing pressure on OTs to define clearly what their role is and their unique contribution to programme planning (Burke, 1984; Kielhofner and Barris, 1984). The key steps in doing this for the forensic population, as for other patient groups, include: (a) stating the philosophy, purpose and goals of OT relevant to the patient population; (b) identifying the needs and characteristics of the population and how they can be addressed by OT; and (c) outlining an operating structure for OT and the procedures to be followed.

Needs of the Population

The range of OT services must be consistent with the needs of the population served by the facility. Therefore, clarification of how the philosophy of OT fits in with the goals of the facility is an important first step. Forensic psychiatric patients have to be treated for their psychiatric condition within a legal framework. The legal framework in itself demands a high degree of accountability on the part of the OT (Lloyd, 1985). It is essential that the OT record the process and outcomes of intervention. The documentation should demonstrate what the therapy is doing and the results obtained (Reed and Sanderson, 1983). The OT is obliged to demonstrate her skills, knowledge and expertise, not only in a clinical context, but in some cases within the courts as well. Treatment, in a criminal justice sense, means helping offenders to avoid further law-breaking (West, 1985). This does not take into account that a significant proportion of these offenders suffer from manifest personal or social deficiencies, or are diagnosed as psychotic, alcohol/drug dependent, sexually deviant, or have anti-social personality disorders and are therefore suitable candidates for psychiatric intervention (West, 1985). The opening of forensic psychiatric facilities with their close links to medical facilities, the courts and university departments of psychiatry, has seen a shift in the care of those individuals who have committed crimes and who have a psychiatric disorder (Freeman, 1982). There is an emphasis on rehabilitative aspects of care rather than on the punitive approach of the correctional/justice system. Treatment resources are now oriented towards those offenders presenting demonstrable problems in coping with their environment (Gendreau, 1985). It has been determined that the forensic patient has three major problem areas which need to be addressed: (a) psychopathology, (b) dysfunction in the performance of their daily occupations, and (c) criminal or anti-social behaviour (Neville, 1980; Freeman, 1982).

An Operating Structure for Occupational Therapy

The health care system requires accountability by demonstrated appropriateness of service. This has a major impact on the OT delivery system (Baum, 1978). The following objectives are considered important in establishing forensic psychiatric OT services:

1 to establish a process of care delivery covering phases of referral, evaluation, treatment planning, delivery of care and termination that is to be followed by all therapists working in the department;
2 to record all patient care according to a standard requiring documentation of evaluation data, recommendations for treatment, a treatment plan with statements of goals and objectives, progress notes and a discharge summary with follow-up recommendations;
3 to require all therapists to apply a relevant frame of reference within which to plan treatment;

4 to require the therapist to carry out formal evaluation to establish both short- and long-term goals before planning individual programmes;
5 to carry out ongoing regular programme evaluation to monitor the effectiveness of the treatment strategies employed.

The Process of Treatment Delivery

Referral

The initial step in the process of treatment is the acquisition of the referral. The referral must come from an authorized source, which within a forensic setting is usually the responsible psychiatrist. Once the referral is received it is necessary to determine its appropriateness and the eligibility of the individual for an OT programme (Hemphill, 1982). Certain key data are required for an acceptable referral (Task Force, 1983). These include: (a) identifying data, i.e., the patient's name, unit, legal status, privilege level; (b) clinical information, i.e., diagnosis, number of previous admissions, reason for current admission, treatment plans, reason for referral; (c) clinical services requested, e.g., activities of daily living assessment, home/personal care training, leisure activities, vocational rehabilitation, social skills; (d) precautions/considerations, e.g., whether impulsive, suicidal, aggressive, or an absconding/elopement risk.

The referral needs to be dated and signed by the responsible psychiatrist and should contain a description of the patient's behaviours or areas of performance which the OT will evaluate. If the referral is appropriate, the OT then undertakes a general assessment of the individual prior to formulating a plan of treatment.

Data Collection

The OT initiates the process of care by data collection. The data base is collected from a variety of sources which may include a review of the patient's progress, consultation with other professionals or community agencies, and from the patient in various ways which may include interview, observation and testing (Task Force, 1983).

The interview is an integral part of the procedure for data collection. The focus is on the individual's functioning in relation to the environment in which he is expected to live. It assists the OT in gaining an understanding of the problems that the individual is experiencing, establishes rapport and involves the individual actively in treatment planning and goal setting. A questionnaire provides a structure for organizing the interview process in order to obtain a profile of the individual which highlights areas of deficits and strengths. At this time the OT decides whether or not further information is necessary. If so, either standardized or non-standardized testing procedures may follow to elaborate on any particular aspect of the patient's functional, cognitive or attitudinal behaviour. We use an activities of daily living questionnaire (copies available on request) that is applicable to a forensic setting as it integrates legal/criminal justice components with the personal data to be gathered.

Evaluation and Treatment

The evaluation process follows data collection and testing procedures. The OT analyses the data, chooses a frame of reference, determines areas of need and draws up a treatment plan based on those identified needs. Re-evaluation is carried out periodically to determine whether or not the patient's needs are being met. The results indicate if the treatment is to continue as planned, or be altered or terminated. The recommendations and the progress of the patient are routinely reported back to the referral source (Hemphill, 1982).

Frames of Reference

A frame of reference is a therapeutic philosophy within which programme planning takes place. The OT identifies a frame of reference — the unique way in which she understands the nature of the patient's problems and in what way they can be effectively remediated (Johnson, 1983). The major theoretical frames of reference that are used within the practice of OT include the humanistic, psychoanalytical, behavioural, developmental, acquisitional, neurodevelopmental, neurobehavioural, spatiotemporal adaptational, occupational behaviour, occupational performance and neurorehabilitation (Llorens, 1984a). It outlines a background mechanism which is based on perceptual, cognitive, psychological and social factors (Reed, 1984). It provides a rationale for understanding the OT process and guides data gathering by suggesting which types of data need collecting. It may also define a range of suitable objectives and how the OT programme may be planned and implemented (Hopkins and Tiffany, 1978; Cubie and Kaplan, 1982). The OT selects from several frames of reference on the basis of patient diagnosis and needs. The resulting programmes therefore may differ for similar patient populations (Creighton, 1985).

In a review of the literature it was found that there has been very little written about the role of OT in forensic psychiatry. It was also found that there were no published articles specifically outlining the frames of reference with specific applicability to a forensic psychiatric population.

Applying an Occupational Behaviour Frame of Reference

For forensic patients many basic skills have never existed or have been lost as a result of institutionalization (Freeman, 1982). In addition, they often experience difficulty in role ability, i.e., the capacity to perform social roles competently (Rogers, 1983a). Successful involvement in occupational functions is seen as a major contributor to mental health and provides structure and meaning to life (Moorhead, 1969). Occupational behaviour is a theoretical framework first described by Reilly (1966). It builds on a sociopsychological definition which regards illness as an impairment of the individual's capacity to perform social roles (Rogers, 1983a). Kielhofner (1983, 1985) has since introduced the model of human occupation which has attempted to synthesize concepts of occupational behaviour into a practice and research model. The basic premise from an occupational behaviour perspective is that individuals spend most of their time occupied in certain types of purposeful activities that occupy time, energy, interest and attention. Throughout the life cycle there is the development of the functions, skills, habits and tasks necessary to engage in occupational roles. This means that there is a recognized sequence in the emergence and execution of such occupying activities as self-maintenance, work and play (Clark, 1979; Kielhofner *et al.*, 1982).

Based on this theoretical viewpoint, a planned OT programme should be directly related to each patient's overall mastery of occupational roles (Clark, 1979). Goals of OT intervention would include directing the patient to: (a) developing habits and practice of skills that improve role performance; (b) adapting occupational behaviour to increase competency in carrying out daily occupations; (c) attaining a balance of occupations necessary for a satisfying and meaningful life; (d) functioning adequately in chosen personal, sexual and occupational roles; and (e) carrying out those occupations which are acceptable to both the individual and society (Clark, 1979; Rogers, 1983a).

An occupational behaviour perspective provides the OT with a framework for assisting the forensic patients to alter their competency in daily occupations. Within this framework interventions are directed towards habit and skill acquisitions which improve role functioning and the quality of life (Rogers, 1983a). It requires that the OT creates a safe and supportive environment within which the patient is helped to identify and practise the skills to carry out the occupational roles which they must fulfil in the community (Cubie and Kaplan, 1982; Clark, 1979).

Remediation through Occupation

Both assessment and treatment are usually equally important functions of forensic service facilities. The evaluation process is defined as using a specific method to measure essential behaviours and provides a clear picture of the patients; of their assets and deficits, and of realistic expectations for future performance (Hopkins and Tiffany, 1978; Rogers, 1983b). Since the OT works as a member of the multidisciplinary team, it is necessary that the OT process integrates with others towards the achievement of the overall treatment objectives for the individual patient. This being the case, it is important that the following basic elements are considered before the setting of short- and long-term goals: (a) the treatment goals and general approach of the multidisciplinary team; (b) the treatment methods and approaches being used by the other team members; (c) the prognosis and clinical management of the patient; (d) the legal status of the patient; (e) the security level appropriate for safe management of the patient; (f) the patient's needs, personal goals and value system; and (g) the occupational roles which they will be expected to carry out in the community (Hopkins and Tiffany, 1978).

When the patient's current status in occupational role performance has been assessed and what needs to be done to enhance occupational performance has been determined, treatment planning can take place (Rogers, 1983b). A treatment plan is a description of the methods and actions that will be used to meet the treatment goals or objectives. Planning is a specific process required to make intervention relevant to the problems and needs of the patient. The treatment programme for a patient in forensic psychiatry, based on an occupational behaviour frame of reference, is organized so that it incorporates the specifications outlined by Reilly (1966). These include:

1 examining the life roles relevant to community adaptation, and identifying the skills to support them and creating an environment whereby the relevant rehabilitative behaviour can be evoked and practised;
2 reflecting the developmental stages present in the acquisition of life skills so that the behaviour can be paced;
3 providing opportunities for natural and legitimate decision-making areas for patients where the skills of successful living can be exercised;

4 providing a milieu which acknowledges competency, arouses curiosity, feeds in universal knowledge, deepens appreciation and demands behaviour — across the full spectrum of an individual's abilities — so that the skills for independent living may be practised;
5 allowing for the work, rest and play aspects of living to be balanced so that the skills pertaining to planning and implementing daily schedules can be acquired;
6 exercising life skills into a balanced pattern of daily living which takes into account interest and ability, and tailors daily events to age, sex and occupational role.

Treatment for the forensic patient should be congruent with the individual's needs, goals, lifestyle and personal and cultural values (Rogers, 1983b). Since it is necessary to prepare the forensic patient with positive personal assets and adaptive skills in specific occupational role/behaviour areas, the OT process is geared towards providing opportunities and experiences that are directly related to improving these skills (Reilly, 1966).

Examples of Treatment Planning Related to Occupational Role

Work performance. Objectives are to (a) increase work tolerance; (b) learn strategies for coping with job stress; (c) learn to carry out task requirements; (d) develop good work habits, e.g., punctuality; (e) learn how to relate to fellow workers; and (f) learn to follow instructions. *Method:* attendance at the workshop where assigned contract work will be carried out.

Vocational preparation. Objectives are to (a) identify employment interests, aptitudes and skills; (b) explore community resources that are available for gathering job information; (c) have the opportunity to fill out an application form and write up a resumé; (d) identify expectations of an employment interview; and (e) investigate potential jobs. *Method:* discussion, pen and paper exercises, role playing, video feedback, visit to the employment agency.

Home management. Objectives are to (a) learn about nutrition; (b) learn how to plan a meal; (c) learn how to shop for meals planned; and (d) learn food preparation and storage. *Method:* discussion, pen and paper exercises, shopping excursions, cooking meals, cleaning up.

Personal care. Objectives are to (a) learn appropriate personal care habits (e.g., regular bathing, cleaning teeth, shaving, cleaning clothes); and (b) learn about clothing maintenance, e.g., washing clothing, ironing, mending. *Method:* watching a film on personal care, keeping a log of personal care routine followed, discussion and practical sessions involving washing and mending clothes.

Leisure planning. Objectives are to (a) identify leisure interests; (b) learn new hobbies, activities and interests; and (c) identify neighbourhood and community interests. *Method:* discussion, pen and paper exercises, craft, sporting activities, visit to community facilities.

Social interaction. Objectives are to (a) learn conversational skills; (b) learn how to be assertive rather than aggressive; (c) identify social activities of interest; (d) learn how to plan social activities; and (e) learn appropriate social skills. *Method:* discussion, pen and paper exercises, role playing, video feedback, involvement in social activities such as bingo, birthday parties, dances.

Community awareness. Objectives are to (a) increase familiarity with local transportation systems; and (b) increase awareness of local community resources. *Method:* trips into the local community with a set agenda and to complete planned exercises.

Case History

George is a 28-year-old single male who was charged with sexual assault and is currently serving a twenty-month sentence that expires in three months' time. He is presently on temporary absence from a correctional facility and has been admitted to the forensic service on a voluntary basis. He has had four previous admissions to hospital. He is diagnosed as anti-social personality disorder and has been treated for his impulsive behaviour which has involved either physical violence or being of a sexual nature. In addition, he has a history of criminal behaviour with charges related to trespassing, possession of a narcotic, trafficking in drugs, and escaping custody.

Educational background. George found school very difficult and did not progress beyond Grade One, spending eight years in special education classes. Some additional courses were commenced but uncompleted.

Employment background. George was 17 when he first began full-time employment. He had held some twenty unskilled jobs, all short-lived and interspersed with either periods of unemployment or incarceration. He had also been fired for exhibiting poor work skills and for laziness. Before being imprisoned, he was working as a farm hand. As he had only been there for a few days, his employer was not interested in his return once released.

Job-seeking skills. George finds it difficult to apply for a job, partly because he does not know how to present himself well at interview, and has difficulties in completing a job application form.

Job behaviour. He also has difficulties in relationships with his co-workers, who tease him because of his poor job skills. In addition, there are problems following orders. He stated: 'If I think a job could be done easier, I get it in my head to do it my way and to hell with what the boss says.' George has many absences from work, because of frequent injuries as well as sometimes simply not feeling like working. He attributes difficulties in carrying out work requirements to low self-esteem, poor work attitude, receiving the minimum wage and having no trade skills. He also frequently oversleeps. When asked if he considered himself a good worker, he replied: 'No. I have no motivation.'

Vocational plans. George would like to work once released but has not made any concrete plans. He desires some vocational training so that he would feel better equipped to look for and obtain work.

Leisure. He likes to spend his leisure time jogging, reading, hiking and swimming, and carries out these activities as often as he can — usually alone, although he does say that he would prefer to do so with other people. He is not familiar with local leisure resources.

Social interaction. George has difficulty making friends and at present he has no close relationships. His family maintains contact with him by writing and telephoning. He is likely to cry when required to talk about how he is not liked and how people 'pick on' him. He has difficulties accepting responsibility for his own behaviour and tends to place blame on such things as birth defects and learning problems. He admits that he can be manipulative when seeking the attention of others, by either being demanding or 'playing the clown'.

Personal and home management. George usually takes care of his hygiene independently. However, when depressed he will go unbathed and unchanged for weeks. Before imprisonment he was living alone in an apartment, and has no firm plans about accommodation when released. His family are not prepared to take him in on a permanent basis. There are further difficulties with meal planning, shopping and cooking; some days he does not bother to eat at all. Usually he exists on such items as packed food and bread and peanut butter. He is unable to balance finances and has trouble paying bills.

Personal qualities/goals. George regards one of his personal qualities as being a caring person. He wishes to improve his self-esteem, improve his living skills, upgrade his education, learn about sexuality and improve his social skills.

Summary. George presents as an insecure man who has many deficits in his general level of functioning in activities of daily living. In terms of his reintegration into the community, George will need a great deal of help with basic self-maintenance skills, work skills and interpersonal skills.

Data Analysis

The data collected provide a baseline of information about the individual. Various areas of functioning are identified as areas of strengths, weaknesses or problems for remediation. The OT organizes a view of the patient from a particular frame of reference and, using the concept of change mechanisms and methods, is able to make recommendations concerning intervention in certain problem areas. As an example, recommendations here would be to improve (a) work skills, (b) money management skills, (c) home management skills, (d) level of personal care, and to (e) develop alternative leisure interests, (f) increase level of community awareness, and (g) improve social interaction skills.

Treatment Plan

The treatment plan is a specific activity required to make intervention relevant to the problems and needs that were identified during the assessment and consistent with the anticipated mechanisms of change. Planning of the OT programme precedes intervention. A treatment plan should improve the following: goals and objectives, i.e., the purpose of the programme and the specific action planned, whether the patient will be seen individually or in groups, the length of time and frequency of sessions, who will carry out the programme, activities chosen, the specific equipment, supplies and facilities required, cost considerations and the frequency, type and method of review (Task Force, 1983). In this case the occupational behaviour frame of reference has been applied. The purpose of the OT programme is to return George to the community with basic self-maintenance skills, improved interpersonal skills and improved work performance skills to equip him for competitive employment. The groups that he will be attending include home management, personal care, work performance, vocational preparation, leisure planning, community awareness and social interaction. Five afternoons per week will be devoted to work performance skills while other groups will involve ninety-minute sessions once per week for eight weeks. With the assistance of therapy assistants the OT will conduct the sessions. Activities will involve such media as pen and paper exercises, films and video in addition to contract work and experiential exercises involving laundry, using the bus, shopping, cooking, etc. Functioning will be reviewed by two methods: a pre-test and a post-test of the groups attended; and a weekly assessment of progress made.

Discussion

Rehabilitation of the forensic psychiatric patient involves focusing on all behaviours that ensure competency in carrying out a social role in the family, on the job and in the community. Changes in the milieu are an important factor for the OT to consider since the interaction between individual differences and the environmental setting can contribute to variance in a patient's behavioural responses and ultimately the treatment outcome (Reilly, 1966; Kannegieter, 1980). The overall aim of the OT programme is to encourage independence and satisfactory performance in all areas of daily living once the patient is returned to the community. To achieve this, the OT needs to focus on the mileu, the evaluation of functional performance and the establishment of goals directed towards maximizing the individual's functional performance. Evaluation of the patient must include an assessment of the functional performance of life tasks and roles in the various environmental settings in which the patient is currently performing and will be expected to perform in the future (Barris, 1982; Howe and Briggs, 1982). In addition, the OT needs to assess the patient's own goals with reference to the changes that they would like to make in carrying out their life tasks and roles. It is these goals which will form the basis of the treatment programme (Howe and Briggs, 1982; Maslen, 1982).

OT is concerned with the interactions of the immediate setting, the social network and the individual, as each individual must interact with these various environmental systems in order to carry out their roles, perform life tasks and to develop life skills. By emphasizing the role of the environment in treatment, patients can be assisted in the development of new appreciations for the environment in their daily interactions (Kannegieter, 1980). The OT needs to facilitate the adaptive process through which an individual may best experience personal life satisfaction (Howe and Briggs, 1982; Kielhofner, 1982 *et al.*, 1982). Thus the environment must provide an optimal level of arousal for each patient. Feedback from the environment enables individuals to monitor and modify responses in order to increase their effectiveness in meeting goals (Kielhofner, 1980). The purposeful activity prescribed by the OT needs to be directly related to the demands of the patient's real life environments. These activities and tasks need to be organized in a sequence where each step must be completed before the patient goes on to the next stage. Sufficient success at each stage gives the individual continuous feedback and encourages him to continue with the activities and tasks (Howe and Briggs, 1982; Maslen, 1982; Llorens, 1984b).

As the aim of the OT programme is to encourage independence and satisfactory performance in all areas of daily living once the patient is returned to the community, the OT needs to consider the total range of occupational behaviour that will be required of the individual in various settings. Since the forensic patient experiences difficulty in carrying out competent occupational role performance, the OT programme needs to emphasize the development of skills and habits. Competency encourages the individual to take a positive role and to increase their repertoire for competent behaviour (Kielhofner, 1980; Barris, 1982; Rogers, 1982). This means that once the patient has mastered the various tasks and roles that are required within the hospital setting, the OT needs to assist the individual in transferring these skills to the community (Heard, 1977; Barris, 1982; Llorens, 1984b).

Conclusions

Occupational therapy is able to contribute significantly to the rehabilitation of the forensic psychiatric patient. This description illustrates a role and contribution based on accurate assessment and treatment planning leading to the development of comprehensive OT programmes for patients seen within this setting. The achievement and maintenance of health and social responsibility as observed in the degree of control that the individual attains over life activities are indications of successful intervention. The greater the person's level of skill in activities that are essential to daily living, the more successful they are likely to be once they return to the community. This being the case, the treatment programme needs to emphasize achievement of competency in the areas of self-care, work, leisure, interactional skills and social role responsibility.

Acknowledgments

With grateful thanks to Antoinette Alleyne, former Supervisor of OT for the Forensic Services, for all the time she spent editing the manuscript; and to Nasir Fiqia, Psychologist for the Forensic Services, for all his assistance in the presentation of the manuscript. This chapter is based on an article published in the *Australian Occupational Therapy Journal,* 34, 1, 1987, 20–5.

References

BARRIS, (1982) 'Environmental interactions: An extension of the model of occupations', *American Journal of Occupational Therapy,* 36, 637–44.

BAUM, (1978) 'Management and documentation of occupational therapy services', in HOPKINS, H. and SMITH, H. (Eds), *Willard and Spackman's Occupational Therapy,* 5th ed., Philadelphia, Pa., J.B. Lippincott Company.

BURKE, J.P. (1984) 'Occupational therapy: A focus for roles in practice'. *American Journal of Occupational Therapy,* 38, 24–8.

CLARKE, P.N. (1979) 'Human development through occupation: A philosophy and conceptual model for practice, part 2', *American Journal of Occupational Therapy,* 33, 577–85.

CREIGHTON, C. (1985) 'Three frames of reference in work related occupational therapy'. *American Journal of Occupational Therapy,* 39, 331–4.

CUBIE, S.H. and KAPLAN, (1982) 'A case analysis method for the model of human occupation', *American Journal of Occupational Therapy,* 36, 465–6.

FREEMAN, M. (1982) 'Forensic psychiatry and related topics', *British Journal of Occupational Therapy,* 45, 191–4.

GENDREAU, P. (1985) 'Critical comments on the practice of clinical criminology', in BEN-ARON, M. *et al.* (Eds), *Clinical Criminology: The Assessment and Treatment of Criminal Behaviour,* Toronto, M and M Graphics.

HEARD, C. (1977) 'Occupational role acquisition', *American Journal of Occupational Therapy,* 31, 243–7.

HEMPHILL, B. (1982) *The Evaluative Process in Psychiatric Occupational Therapy,* Thorofare. N.J., Charles B. Slack.

HOPKINS, H. and TIFFANY, E. (1978) 'Occupational therapy: A problem solving process', in HOPKINS, H. and SMITH, H., (Eds), *Willard and Spackman's Occupational Therapy,* 5th ed., Philadelphia, Pa., J.B. Lippincott Company.

HOWE, M. and BRIGGS, A. (1982) 'Ecological systems model for occupational therapy', *American Journal of Occupational Therapy,* 36, 322–7.

JOHNSON, J. (1983) 'The changing medical marketplace as a context for the practice of occupational therapy', in KIELHOFNER, G., (Ed.), *Health through Occupation: Theory and Practice in Occupational Therapy,* Philadelphia, Pa., F.A. Davis Company.

KANNEGIETER, R. (1980) 'Environmental interactions in psychiatric occupational therapy — some inferences', *American Journal of Occupational Therapy,* 34, 715–20.

KIELHOFNER, G. (1980) 'A model of human occupation, part 3: Benign and vicious cycles', *American Journal of Occupational Therapy* , 34, 715–20.

KIELHOFNER, G. (1982) 'A heritage of activity: Development of theory', *American Journal of Occupational Therapy,* 36, 20–21.

KIELHOFNER, G. (1983) *Health through occupation: Theory and Practice in Occupational Therapy,* Philadelphia, Pa., F.A. Davis Company.

KIELHOFNER, G. (1985) *A Model of Human Occupation: Theory and Application,* Baltimore, Md., Williams and Wilkins.

KIELHOFNER, G. and BARRIS, R. (1984) 'Mental health occupational therapy: Trends in literature and practice', *Occupational Therapy in Mental Health,* 4, 35–51.

KIELHOFNER, G., BURKE, J. and IGI, C. (1980) 'A model of human occupation, part 4: Assessment and intervention', *American Journal of Occupational Therapy,* 34, 777–88.

KIELHOFNER, G., BARRIS, R. and WATTS, J.H. (1982) 'Habits and habit dysfunction: A clinical perspective for psychological occupational therapy', *Occupational Therapy in Mental Health,* 2, 723–30.

LLORENS, L. (1984a) 'Theoretical conceptualizations of occupational therapy: 1960–1982', *Occupational Therapy in Mental Health,* 4, 1–14.

LLORENS, L. (1984b) 'Changing balance: Environment and individual', *American Journal of Occupational Therapy,* 38, 29–34.

LLOYD, C. (1985) 'Evaluation and forensic psychiatric occupational therapy', *British Journal of Occupational Therapy,* 48, 137–40.

MASLEN, D. (1982) 'Rehabilitation training for community living skills: Concepts and techniques', *Occupational Therapy in Mental Health,* 2, 33–49.

MOORHEAD, L. (1969) 'The occupational history', *American Journal of Occupational Therapy,* 23, 329–34.

NEVILLE, A. (1980) 'Temporal adaptation: Application with short-term psychiatric patients. *American Journal of Occupational Therapy,* 34, 328–31.

REED, K. (1984) *Models of Practice in Occupational Therapy,* Baltimore, Md., Willians and Wilkins.

REED, K. and SANDERSON, S. (1983) *Concepts of Occupational Therapy,* 2nd ed., Baltimore, Md., Williams and Wilkins.

REILLY, M. (1966) 'A psychiatric occupational therapy program as a teaching model', *American Journal of Occupational Therapy,* 20, 61–7.

RICE, M. (1985) 'Violence in a maximum security hospital: A researcher-clinician's perspective', in BEN-ARON, M. *et al.* (Eds), *Clinical Criminology: The Assessment and Treatment of Criminal Behaviour,* Toronto, M and M Graphics.

ROGERS, J. (1982) 'The spirit of independence: The evolution of a philosophy', *American Journal of Occupational Therapy,* 36, 709–15.

ROGERS, J. (1983a) 'The study of human occupation', in KIELHOFNER, G. (Ed.), *Health through Occupation: Theory and Practice in Occupational Therapy,* Philadelphia, Pa., F.A. Davis Company.

ROGERS, J. (1983b) 'Clinical reasoning: The ethics, science and art', *American Journal of Occupational Therapy*, 37, 601–16.

SMITH, S. (1984) 'The forensic model of occupational therapy', *Occupational Therapy in Mental Health*, 4, 17–23.

TASK FORCE (1983) *Guidelines for the Client-centred Practice of Occupational Therapy*, Ottawa, Ministry of National Health and Welfare.

WEST, D. (1985) 'Clinical criminology under attack', in BEN-ARON, M. *et al.* (Eds), *Clinical Criminology: The Assessment and Treatment of Criminal Behaviour*, Toronto, M and M Graphics.

Chapter 15

Treatment of Substance Abuse and Alcoholism

Barbara Konkol and Mary Jo Schneider

In the area of chemical dependency and alcoholism the OT is effectively able to focus attention on the integration on the many aspects of daily living skills and the application of these skills to individual life situations. Occupational therapy services in the treatment of chemical dependency and alcoholism combine a knowledge of physical and psychosocial dysfunction.

Problems

Physical Problems

Alcohol is absorbed into the blood primarily from the small intestine. The principal effect of alcohol is depression of the central nervous system (CNS). Depending on the amount ingested, alcohol produces sedation or tranquility, lack of coordination and intoxication and, with large amounts, unconsciousness. People who drink large amounts of alcohol typically become somewhat tolerant of its effects. Those tolerant to alcohol are often also tolerant to many other CNS depressants such as barbiturates and benzodiazepines. The physical dependence accompanying tolerance is profound and withdrawal produces a series of adverse effects that may lead to death (Berkow, 1982). The adverse effects of mild alcohol withdrawal include tremor, weakness, sweating and gastrointestinal symptoms. As withdrawal becomes more diffuse, some patients may suffer grande mal seizures. Delerium tremens (DTs), the most severe type of alcohol withdrawal, begin with anxiety attacks, increasing confusion, poor sleep, marked sweating and depression. As the condition worsens, hallucinations may occur. The person may then experience a coarse tremor of the hands which can extend to the head and trunk. The mortality of DTs may be as high as 15 per cent (Berkow, 1982).

The biological and physiological problems associated with alcoholism and chemical dependency have a devastating effect on the body's ability to maintain homeostasis. This is supported by the fact that alcohol may cause damage to almost every organ in the body (AIMS Media, 1984). Cirrhosis of the liver, cardiomyopathy, esophageal varices, peripheral neuropathy, increased rates of lung and throat cancer, and decreased sex drive are frequently associated with alcohol abuse. In general, a decrease in the level of overall strength and endurance can be noted in individuals who have been abusing alcohol and/or drugs.

Psychological Problems

Cognitive problems are perhaps the most evident. Disorientation in time, place and person is common. Short-term and long-term memory lapses may exist due to blackouts. Many individuals confabulate incidents in an attempt to compensate for memory problems. Perceptual deficits with regard to size, shape, colour and visual memory hinder performance of daily living skills and structured tasks. Damage to the cerebrum often results in decreased judgment, problem-solving and decision-making abilities. Maladaptive behaviours also occur due to increased alcohol/drug ingestion. These behaviours include aggressiveness, loquacity, irritability, euphoria, depression and emotional lability. In severe cases patients may develop organic brain syndrome. Korsakoff's psychosis is a type of organic brain syndrome characterized by a severe impairment in memory. The syndrome is also called 'Wernicke's Korsakoff' because the condition is manifested by difficulty in comprehending and encoding new information (Lezak, 1983). Behavioural defects associated with Korsakoff's psychosis are disorientation for time and place, loss of initiative, disinterest, irritability, anger or pleasure. Lezak reported that these defects may quickly dissipate when the stimulating condition is removed or the discussion topic is changed. The etiology of Koraskoff's syndrome has been attributed to thiamine deficiency. Baum and Iber (1984) concluded that alcoholism interferes with the absorption of thiamine which directly affects the CNS. The syndrome, however, may also be found in patients with poor dietary intake and no history of alcoholism . Some patients show improvements in memory when treated with vitamin therapy.

As the disease of chemical dependency progresses, individuals experience a decreased self-esteem along with frequent feeling of self-pity, hopelessness and helplessness. Such feelings are complicated when an individual uses defence mechanisms to explain their addiction. Denial is the most prominent defence used by chemically dependent individuals. The denial manifests itself in three common forms: (a) denial of the alcoholism and/or chemical dependency; (b) denial of the need for rehabilitation or long-term treatment; and (c) denial of physical, social and psychological problems secondary to chemical abuse. Minimization is recognized when the patient verbalizes a lack of bio-psychosocial problems associated with chemical dependency. Further minimization is observed when clients report ingesting their drug of choice in decreased quantity and frequency in contrast to their medical history. Rationalization is another defence mechanism used in an attempt to justify addiction and make it appear socially acceptable. Common rationalizations include drinking due to marriage problems, job stress, loneliness, boredom, peer pressure and health problems. While many individuals that enter treatment have suffered legitimate losses such as death of a spouse or child, or loss of a job, it is necessary to reinforce the fact that drinking and/or drug use is an inappropriate method of coping with such losses. Intellectualization becomes apparent when clients verbalize/analyze problems secondary to chemical dependency without revealing feelings and emotions. It has been noted that intellectualization increases with an individual's level of education and is consequently more prevalent amongst impaired professionals.

Social Problems

Further impairment arises in the area of social-interpersonal development. The chemically dependent individual encounters strained relationships with significant others in the home as well as in the workplace. Prolonged abuse often leads to loss of employment and associated financial problems which add further strain to family relationships.

Many problems are found in the family. Due to prolonged resentments, fear of being alone and unresolved grief, the spouse may insidiously sabotage the chemical abuser's attempts to maintain sobriety. On other occasions the spouse has experienced so many broken promises that he/she is cynical and doubting. Also the presence of an alcoholic parent can be very destructive to the self-esteem of the children as they see their adult role model flawed. It is not surprising that the divorce rate is higher in chemically dependent families.

Young abusers often quit pursuing their education in an effort to find employment to support their habit. Financial problems may become legal in nature as abusers succumb to crime in order to subsidize their addiction. Other legal problems may include driving a motor vehicle under the influence of alcohol and/or drugs as well as disorderly conduct charges.

Aspects of Therapy

Evaluation

The OT works in a variety of settings with the chemically dependent individual. These settings are both public and private and include outpatient clinics, half-way houses, acute-care hospitals and extended-care treatment centres. Regardless of the type of setting, the OT works in close conjunction with a multidisciplinary treatment team usually consisting of a physician, and alcohol and other drug abuse (AODA) counsellor, nurse, dietician, physiotherapist and activity therapist. Since chemically dependent clients are often manipulative and controlling, it is important to maintain an open line of communication with team members so that disruptive behaviours can be confronted in an appropriate manner. Good communication between members further ensures that a client's needs will be met in a prompt and effective manner.

Once the OT becomes familiar with the disease concept of chemical dependency and associated bio-psychosocial problems and behaviours, she is ready to establish contact with the client. This contact is often established during the initial evaluation.

There is no standardized OT evaluation for assessing chemically dependent clients. Since the chemically dependent individual may present with multiple problems (physical, psychological and social), the initial evaluation needs to assess all of these areas. This initial evaluation should begin with an explanation of the facility's OT programme and its relevance to the recovery process. Following this explanation, it is helpful for the OT to gather a brief psychosocial history so each patient may be treated as a unique individual. Gathering the history through a verbal question and answer format, the OT has an opportunity to assess the client's perception of the disease and associated bio-psychosocial problems. For example, do the patients use defence mechanisms to explain their addiction? Are they accurate historians? The history may further reveal potential obstacles to the client's recovery such as decreased motivation, a history of relapse or extensive health problems.

A self-evaluation may be used to assist the clients in identification of feelings and behaviours related to their addictions. In addiction, feelings related to self-esteem are identified. The self-evaluation may be utilized as a means to assess strengths, weaknesses and perceptions of one's abilities. The OT may use a separate goal list to identify problems that need to be addressed throughout treatment. Such a list would further clarify the client's perception of alcohol and drug-related problems.

A method used to establish a baseline on the client's mental and abstract age is the Shipley Institute of Living Scale. These tests measure 'the extent to which the individual's abstract thinking falls short of his vocabulary' (Shipley-Boyle, 1967).

At some treatment facilities the client may be placed in a specific rehabilitation group following the completion of all evaluations. These rehabilitation groups are comprised of peers with similar age, diagnosis and level of cognitive function. It has been found that placing individuals amongst peers with similar needs will decrease initial stress and anxiety as well as promote a sense of support within the group.

Occupational therapy goals with the chemically dependent population focus on increasing the clients' self-awareness of how substance abuse has altered their values, actions, physical status and emotional state. Throughout treatment emphasis is placed of assisting clients to resume previous levels of daily life management as well as improving judgment and safety procedures in functional task performance (Occupational Therapy Association of California, 1979). Goals are accomplished by participation in discussion and task groups. The most important goal is for clients to take an active role in their treatment because recovery is a continuous and active process. The active role assures that clients are assuming responsibility for their actions to improve their daily living skills as well as the social and interpersonal skills needed to facilitate maintained sobriety. Once these skills are perfected in the treatment setting, they can be applied to specific areas such as employment and education.

Treatment

Occupational therapy treatment of chemically dependent individuals parallels Mosey's acquisitional frame of reference which 'focuses upon the various skills or abilities which the individual needs for adequate and satisfying interaction in the environment' (Mosey, 1977, p. 17). In general, alcohol and substance abusers need to develop improved social, leisure and stress management skills. According to Mosey, 'it is further assumed that corrective learning experiences will lead to acquisition of desirable abilities and thus allow the individual to continue the process of self-actualization' (Mosey, 1977, p. 17). The OT group provides an excellent environment in which corrective learning experiences may take place. The OT needs to encourage clients to accept responsibility for their actions and identify and clarify values in order to make the necessary changes in lifestyle to maintain sobriety. Once sober, individuals can re-establish a focus on becoming more self-actualized individuals. Within OT practice Katz (1985) defines 'human occupation as the core of the domain of concern.' In this category Katz includes 'daily living tasks, work, play, recreation and leisure'. Alcohol and drug abusers need to place emphasis in these areas for a variety of reasons. For example, clients often neglect personal hygiene and overall appearance when using alcohol and drugs. Nutritional intake suffers as alcohol fills an individual with 'empty calories', and many drugs decrease appetite. Overall job performance suffers due to lack of concentration, alertness and/or poor attendance. Many individuals need to relearn responsibility and follow through with simple tasks so that these behaviours may be assimilated to a work setting. For many clients social recreation may have centred on use of alcohol/drugs in a public place or social atmosphere, while others may have abused substances alone and at home. Regardless of the situation, alcohol and drug abusers simply lack awareness, motivation and insight to change behaviours associated with substance abuse. This includes finding new leisure interests as well as a new peer group with whom they can associate.

Katz (1985) further identified the 'competence components of sensory integration, neuromuscular function, cognitive function, psychological function and social interaction' (p. 521) as parameters of OT practice. The subjects of psychological functioning and well-being require major emphasis during OT discussion groups. The OT can encourage clients to identify and express internalized feelings that have been repressed while using various substances. The OT utilizes structured task projects to assist clients in increasing a sense of self-esteem through taking pride in finished products. This is an important factor as chemically dependent individuals are noted for procrastinating when plans or projects need to be completed. In addition, working with less structured tasks allows clients to develop an improved frustration tolerance and decreased need for immediate gratification. Stress management focuses on the development of appropriate coping skills for use in anxiety provoking situations. The OT may provide biofeedback training or other relaxation techniques as a form of stress management (see Chapter 10). This is an important area of emphasis since clients are accustomed to seeking chemical relief for stress. The OT can assist clients in identifying individual life stressors and coping skills which they can practise before discharge. Occupational therapy assertiveness groups provide clients with the opportunity to practise making requests and refusals without feeling guilty. During assertiveness groups the client may also practise verabalizing anger and related negative feelings in a non-aggressive manner. Exercises in values clarification assist clients in setting priorities by identifying values and behaviours that need to be changed to facilitate maintenance of a drug-free lifestyle. The topic of lifestyle change should include increased emphasis on identification and implementation of needed alterations since many clients are 'treatment wise' and put more emphasis on verbalization of change than actual follow-through.

The OT can facilitate the competence component of social interaction by encouraging peers to mingle with each other during group discussion and task behaviour. In addition, the OT can direct group members to take risks involving initiating conversations with other staff and peers not directly involved in their treatment group. This is extremely important since many clients isolate themselves and become engrossed in self-pity to the extent that they believe they can recover on their own. Nonetheless, it has been shown that 'tendencies towards loneliness' and 'irritation with friends' are two relapse warning signs (Miller *et al.*, 1982).

Cognitive functioning as a competence component is addressed through participation in current events groups. Clients are motivated to discuss trends and topics of prevailing interest. This approach is less demeaning and more intellectually challenging than having clients simply identify the day, date, month and year. Memory and decision-making are monitored during task behaviour as clients complete projects suited to their level of cognitive capabilities.

The sensory integration and neuromuscular competence components as defined by Katz can be applied to clients who are diagnosed with peripheral neuropathy secondary to alcohol abuse. Strengthening and sensory input are used to promote the restoration of sensory-motor function.

Occupational therapists may further treat the chemically dependent patient on a behavioural basis if additional emphasis is needed in the area previously mentioned. Working in this manner gives the therapist more time to focus on individual problems which the client may be experiencing. Time management and goal setting are two areas frequently addressed in these sessions. Since many chemically dependent individuals have spent the majority of their time being non-productive, it is paramount that they learn how to budget time in a constructive manner. Further emphasis on goal setting ensures that clients choose goals which are realistic as well as within their means of accomplishment.

Ongoing Assessment

As treatment progresses, assessment of patient performance becomes an ongoing, continuous process. Observation of behaviour is the primary means of assessment. Treatment plans need to be individualized for each client. The OT needs to provide measurable, realistic goals in which the patient can demonstrate methods of follow-through and completion. Any change noted in the core area of human occupational or competence components should be documented so other team members are aware of progress or setbacks. Effective communication with treatment team members is essential since substance abusers often engage in manipulation of staff.

Manipulative behaviour and negative attitudes are two obstacles which the OT working with the chemically dependent population will encounter. Resistance to treatment in the form of poor attendance and unwillingness to become an active group member is also common. It is the duty of the therapist to confront clients with this type of behaviour and remind them that the benefits derived from treatment are equal to the amount of effort exerted in the recovery process.

Emphasis in treatment is placed on doing. Fidler and Fidler (1978) define doing as 'enabling the development and integration of the sensory, motor, cognitive and psychological systems; serving as a socializing agent, and verifying one's efficacy as a competent, contributing member of one's society' (p. 305). If clients maintain an active role in their treatment, they are accepting responsibility to become more productive members in society and self-actualized human beings.

Discharge and After-care

The OT assists the patient in preparation for discharge by addressing specific competence components necessary to perform daily living tasks. For example, the OT may assess vocational readiness. This can be accomplished by role playing or videotaping a simulated job interview session. The OT may also assist the client with compiling a resumé as well as reviewing public job postings. Other areas addressed in preparation for discharge include budgetting skills, identifying community resources for leisure pursuits, teaching awareness of nutritional needs, food shopping and cooking, and use of public transportation.

The need for ongoing treatment and support for the chemically dependent individual cannot be overemphasized. The rehabilitation of the patient frequently breaks down as soon as they leave the treatment facility. Time spent in treatment represents only a small fraction of total life. Follow-up studies tend to demonstrate that the substance abuser's continued deterioration is usually associated with a lack of close interpersonal relationships with family or friends (Fink *et al.*, 1985). Therefore, in preparation for discharge a concerted effort must be made to re-establish sociological balance.

There are many agencies and organizations concerned with chemical dependency which provide resources and support. Alcoholics Anonymous and Drugs Anonymous (DA) are self-help groups whose basic aim is to bring members to help each other achieve and maintain a chemically free lifestyle. Much effort has been devoted to explaining and understanding these organizations' accomplishments, significance and meaning. Some view the programmes as a resocialization process promoting individual maturation through the member's assumption of increased responsibility, first to themselves and then to others. Some assert that it helps each member achieve a new self-concept in which the need for outside assistance is recognized as acceptable and vital. Whatever the reasons for success, these organizations have been extremely valuable to innumerable people.

Self-help groups are available for the family, friends and children of chemically dependent individuals. In addition, there are programmes sponsored by religious organizations, industrial and labour union programmes, public health centres and schools.

Conclusions

In conclusion, the role of the OT in working with the chemically dependent population is threefold. Firstly, she serves as an educator, teaching clients about human occupation and associated competence components. Secondly, she serves as a facilitator to increase patient awareness of the lifestyle changes necessary in order to maintain sobriety. Thirdly, she is a monitor who observes, recognizes and confronts clients with typical addictive behaviours.

References

AIMS MEDIA (1984) 'Alcohol and Human Physiology', film, California, Van Nuys.

BAUM, R. and IBER, F. (1984) 'Thiamin — the interaction of aging, alcoholism, and malabsorption in various populations', *World Review of Nutritional Dietetics*, 44, 85–116.

BERKOW, R. (1982) *The Merck Manual*, 14th ed., New Jersey, Merck, Sharp and Dohme Research Labs.

FIDLER, G. and FIDLER, J. (1978) 'Doing and becoming: Purposeful action and self-actualization', *American Journal of Occupational Therapy*, 32, 305–10.

FINK, A., LONGABAUGH, R., MCCRADY, B., STOUT, R., BEATTIE, M., RUGGIERI-AUTHELET, A. and MCNEIL, D. (1985) 'Effectiveness of alcoholism treatment in partial versus inpatient settings', *Addictive Behaviours*, 10, 235–48.

KATZ, N. (1985) 'Occupational therapy's domain of concern: Reconsidered', *American Journal of Occupational Therapy*, 39, 518–24.

LEZAK, M.D. (1983) *Neuropsychological Assessment*, New York, Oxford University Press.

MILLER, M., ORSKI, T. and MILLER, D. (1982) *Learning to Live Again: A Guide for Recovery from Alcoholism*, 3rd ed., Missouri, Independence Press.

MOSEY, A. (1977) *Three Frames of Reference for Mental Health*, Thorofare, N.J., Charles B. Slack.

OCCUPATIONAL THERAPY ASSOCIATION OF CALIFORNIA (1979) *Occupational Therapy Practice Guidlines*, Calif., Occupational Therapy Association of California.

SHIPLEY-BOYLE, B. (1967) *The Shipley Institute of Living Scale,* Hartford, Conn., The Institute of Living.

Chapter 16

Occupational Therapy with Eating Disorders

Rose Stockwell, Sheena Duncan and Mary Levens

This chapter aims to tune the potential therapist's mind into some of the areas which may be worth considering before embarking on therapy within eating disorders. It does not attempt to be encompassing, but merely to give some theoretical background and highlight potential difficulties. It is recognized that methods of practice rely on a growing body of systematic knowledge. However, the need for therapists to combine this knowledge with carefully supervized work is emphasized. Stern (1986) has pointed out the disadvantages of 'doing things by the book': '. . . there is the danger with any prescribed approach that it will be applied in a mechanical way, thus running the risk of repeating one of the major traumas of the anorexic and bulimic families; a rigid, mechanical approach to child rearing that does not take into account the child's unique and shifting needs.'

The Relationship between Therapist and Patient

As well as testing the system as a whole, the therapist needs to be aware of the specific relationship developed with the patient. The issues can be complex, and therapists are recommended to obtain supervision for their work with these patients. The need for the therapist to have personal awareness and self-understanding has been emphasized by various writers. Barr (1980) suggests that to create a successful therapeutic relationship one needs to be aware of one's personality and prejudices. We need to recognize why we like some people and not others, recognize that certain sayings, theories or gestures will annoy us and not others, and generally try to understand how we 'tick' so that we can better understand our relationships with other people. To paraphrase Furnham *et al.* (1980), a good relationship between the OT and patient contributes fundamentally to the effectiveness of treatment. Indeed, the quality of the relationship can often determine the duration and course of the readoption process. Establishing rapport consists of starting and maintaining a relationship in which free, honest supportive communication can flourish. Communication is a two-way process but responsibility for it must inevitably rest with the OT as the helping professional. The therapist will often teach communication skills unwittingly, by example rather than formally, and so it is important that her example be a good one. Casement (1985) reminds us that although there are many different caring professions, the psychodynamics of any helping relationship may be universal. Therefore, it is important to become familiar with the ways in which 'helper' and 'client' interact and communicate with each other.

The specific areas of personal awareness and self-understanding that therapists working with eating disordered people need to consider include their own eating patterns; how they feel about their own weight; how they feel about their own shape; and whether they will be able to respond non-defensively in these areas. One reason for examining these specific areas is that a patient may enquire of the therapist if they themselves have had an eating problem. Therapists must have an answer to this question which reflects their own position and indicates their level of understanding and empathy. It is considered normal in our society for weight and shape to be a sensitive area for women. Therapists need to be sure, however, that their personal interest is not exaggerating the patient's problem. If a therapist responds defensively to an area which is personally difficult, the patient may 'look after' the therapist by leaving the topic alone or, alternatively, talk extensively about the topic as if to help 'sort out' the therapist! Experienced therapists use their supervision time for identifying areas which are personally difficult. The therapist, just like the patient, can become a better person and a better therapist by recognizing their defensive behaviours and understanding the underlying conflicts that lead them to respond in this way.

There are many issues which underlie a person's eating disorder, but some which regularly emerge include the following: (a) separation, which includes leaving home, ending a relationship and being adopted; (b) loss, which includes deaths of family or friends which are not grieved sufficiently, and loss of friends through parents separating or the family moving to a new area; (c) dealing with parental conflict, which includes needing to act as pacifier or go-between; and (d) breaking away from parental social expectations.

Where therapists find a parallel between the patient's problems and their own, they need to be sensitive to their potential to confuse the two. In addition, there will be feelings which the patient has about the therapist. These may include jealousy, rage and envy. The patient will often see the therapist as a competent person successfully coping with a job, food and their social and personal relationships. The therapist needs to be able to accept these feelings from the patient and examine how such feelings affect the therapeutic relationship and then broaden these to the patient's current and past relationships. Davenloo (1980) suggests that these links are very important. Basically the therapist actively works on two psychodynamic 'triangles'. Firstly, there is the triangle of conflict: defences (D) — anxiety (A) — impulse-feeling (I–F). Secondly, there is the triangle of person: transference (T) — significant people in the patient's current life (C) — significant people in the past (P). The crucial part of the technique consists of making the links in the second triangle, especially in pointing out the parallels between the patient's reactions to the transference and current people (the T–C link) and between the transference and the past (the T–P link). The second triangle is completed when all three possible links are made (the T–C–P link). The prognosis is definitely better and the length of treatment definitely shorter, the sooner and more often a T–P or T–C–P interpretation can be made in a meaningful way (Davenloo, 1980). As part of treatment, the patient's loss of symptoms may coincide with intense feelings of anger and depression. The therapist needs to tolerate these feelings without being overwhelmed and to facilitate the patient's ability to bear such feelings without returning to binging.

Treatments for Eating Disorders

Individuals coming for treatment have learned maladaptive ways of coping with a variety of situations and emotions and the therapist's role is to facilitate modification of these coping skills. Young (1984) refers to four characteristics of individual adaptation: (a) the individual is active, not passive, in the process; (b) environmental demands or needs, tasks and goals evoke the adaptive response; (c) this adaptive response is organized at a subcortical level, while the individual's attention is directed to the activity (task); and (d) successful responses feed back as reinforcers to meet the next challenge. Most treatments follow these stages; many reinforce the subcortical process with activities aimed at making the individual conscious of their behaviour, and most stress the importance of the patient taking responsibility for the progress which they make and for the skills developed. In all treatments therapists respect the patient's rights and individuality, do not impose attitudes or prejudices, and are responsible for encouraging and facilitating the self-realization of the patient. Therapists work to help the patient increase the range of choices open to them and their powers to make decisions.

Treatment of Anorexia Nervosa

Treatment occurs mainly within an inpatient setting. Outpatient treatment consists of individual counselling, family therapy and/or group treatment and is used to facilitate a natural recovery, as part of the discharge plan for those for whom the inpatient treatment is unsuitable or as a step towards admission.

Inpatient treatment of anorexia nervosa (AN). Most team approaches combine a behavioural programme aimed at establishing normal eating behaviour and a psychodynamic approach aimed at helping the patient come to a greater understanding of themselves and working towards increased autonomy and individualization. A typical programme is summarized next (Crisp *et al.*, 1985).

During the initial stages or 'refeeding' the aim is to increase the weight of the patient. Each patient will have a specific 'target weight', the calculation of which is dependent on the patient's age when AN commenced, their build and height. In the early stages of the refeeding programme the patient can be resistant to interventions, hiding food, exercising on her bed and generally 'holding back' from staff. These actions can contribute to the staff feeling angry and unsympathetic towards the patient. Additionally many patients at their lowest weight are dissociated from their emotional world due to their starvation state and are wholly concerned about food. This limits areas of treatment which the patient can be involved in and the staff need to work closely together. As described by Stern (1986), in the refeeding programme staff need to be supportive and empathic yet firm. Initially they need to take over responsibility for the refeeding process and then transfer their responsibility back to the patient.

Following this first stage of treatment, the anorexic patient has significant development tasks to face if her symptoms are to be surrendered. Crisp's view is that the therapeutic position is that the anorexic is being asked to trade in her AN (essentially her avoidance stance) for the ultimate prospect of full recovery. She is invited to surrender her spurious and only current freedom (to sustain her AN) in return for the potential freedom inherent in gaining weight and in thereby rediscovering her mature self and expressing it in a healthier manner. She will need to experience this as acceptable and sufficiently fulfilling and that others will anticipate that she will have considerable emotional problems in this respect for somewhile (perhaps years). Furthermore, she needs to know that the potential for redeveloping AN is quite possible. The OT needs to be aware of this somewhat gloomy prognosis for many patients with AN and to keep treatment goals realistic. It may also be of help to consider the classification of subgroups of AN by Stern when considering OT aims and objectives and choice of activities. This author suggests that three subgroups of 'the borderline', 'the empty, understructured' and 'the emotionally-conflicted, identify confused' form a continuum of difficulties related to the patient's capacity for separation/individuation.

Occupational Therapy with Inpatient Anorexics

Assessment. Assessment should include (a) motivation to change (eating patterns and coping strategies); (b) a degree of insight into self and into the consequences and effects of her behaviour; (c) attention and concentration span; (d) personal interests and talents; (e) feelings about the family; (f) school or work situation; and (g) social and family life.

Early stages of treatment. At this stage activities will be limited due to low weight, the patient being restricted to bed-rest and possibly also due to having an emotional 'switch off'. The main aim is to develop a secure therapeutic relationship which lays the foundation for future treatment activities where the patient will be risking experiencing and expressing denied feelings and needs. The therapist may share some personal experiences and feelings with the patient as a model of expressing positive and negative feelings, doubts and uncertainties, happiness and confidence.

The patient's aims may include being spontaneous, developing self-expression, learning to take appropriate control in situations and being able to make decisions based on assessing pros and cons of situations.

Activities which are used include art and clay work which also provide a medium for the ventilation of feelings. Where themes are used, the therapist may make suggestions initially but would aim to hand over initiative to the patient. The therapist may join in sometimes to promote spontaneity and enjoyment. Where art takes place in a group, the therapist will be encouraging the development of the patient's sense of individuality and the recognition of shared areas of identification with others. Difficulties which the therapist may anticipate include the patient feeling that their work is 'not good enough', seeking continuous reassurance, needing to feel that their time is being spent productively, and needing structure and organization.

Treatment in the middle stages. Further aims may be included at this stage such as modifying body image, acceptance of body shape, developing awareness, gaining new social and assertive skills, showing initiative and learning anxiety management. Activities used to facilitate these aims include relaxation, assertion, communication skills, psychodrama, movement therapy, craft activities and creative writing. The difficulties which may emerge now include extreme disgust towards their new size and shape, mixing exclusively with other patients with AN, making comparisons of themselves with others, competitiveness, and witholding their feelings from others. Activities which require mixing, an exchange of personal qualities and confrontration, are applicable.

Relaxation increases body awareness and may evoke panic feelings which lead either to increased tension or to a need to increase control in other areas, e.g., food. The therapist should explore these difficulties with the patient. Psychodrama helps patients discover and develop new aspects of themselves which in turn help them to cease AN. Enacting relationship difficulties and personal conflicts allows family interactions to be examined and can highlight themes of family therapy. Bruch (1978) maintains that the crux of treatment is the resolution of the patient's feelings about their bodies, and movement therapy promotes this resolution. Movement is usually introduced towards the end of this stage. Physical activities (e.g., swimming) may have been used as part of the person's way of sustaining weight loss and they may be tempted to abuse such again. In treatment firm boundaries are set and the amount of physical exercise is built up slowly to ensure that weight loss does not occur.

Treatment in the latter stages. Additional aims to be added later include planning and cooking meals, eating with others, and work, school and career issues.

Dealing with the practicalities of food is a sensitive but crucial area usually undertaken in the latter stages of treatment. At first the patient may cook a simple meal with the therapist and spend time talking about the difficulties of doing this. They may initially need to plan appropriately balanced meals and shop together. The patient may be tempted to old habits such as avoiding sugars and fats in recipes and choosing low calorie products. Gradually the patient will cook more difficult meals and eat with others. They may invite their partner or family for several meals before leaving hospital. Finally, eating in public places, such as a restaurant, may be added.

Work and school problems revolve around the issues identified earlier in treatment such as the patient striving to be perfect in her studies or employment and being overconscientious. At this stage the therapist provides as many realistic opportunities as possible for the patient to try new ways of behaving. Some employers and schools may be willing to allow the person to go back for trial days which can then be discussed with the therapist.

Treatment of Bulimia Nervosa (BN)

Initial assessment. Unlike AN, BN may be successfully treated in both inpatient and outpatient settings. The initial assessment is used to identify which treatment setting is appropriate for an individual. Aronson (1986) and Lacey (1985) have both described similar subgroupings for BN. Aronson's 'low level bulimics' are equivalent to Lacey's 'personality disordered group' and Aronson's 'high level group' are equivalent to Lacey's 'neurotic group'. Thus patients with BN range from low level/personality disordered to high level/neurotic patients. Those tending towards the lower end require inpatient treatment, while those tending towards the higher end are treated in outpatient programmes.

The low level/personality disordered group. The low level bulimic's life is characterized by chronic binging and daily vomiting. The person feels like a helpless victim of a mysterious disease and can rarely identify precipitants. Poor reality testing is shown by the life threatening behaviour of the extensive vomiting, uses of laxatives and starvation (Aronson, 1986). In the personality disordererd group manipulation of food is associated to a varying degree with alcohol and drug abuse. Clinically such patients present as emotionally shallow or histrionic. Overdosing and superficial wrist cutting are not infrequent (Lacey, 1985).

The high level neurotic group. Binging and vomiting are less frequent in this group, and there may be no vomiting at all. There may be periods of normal eating, but binging and vomiting are turned to in response to stress, rejection and disappointment. The capacity for delayed gratification is somewhat more so in these patients. Addictive behaviours such as smoking and drinking are frequent too, although they are less likely to drink excessively at any one time than the lower level group (Aronson, 1986). The patients tend to be hard working and ambitious with high ethical standards. The predominant clinical symptom, apart from the eating disorder, is anger, although often initially denied. Feelings of sadness or depression are more likely to be described readily and on deeper examination low self-esteem and a feeling of being a failure will also be admitted. Presentation at a clinic is usually precipitated by emotional distress associated with relationship difficulties (Lacey, 1985).

Positive indicators for outpatient treatment. In addition to meeting the general description of a higher level patient, the following are a few features which are positive indicators for outpatient treatment: (a) they sought treatment for themselves; (b) they are not suicidal; (c) they will accept maintaining their weight within the normal range; and (d) they wish to change their attitudes and eating habits.

Treatment Methods

All treatments aim to stop patients binging and purging, and to help them feel sufficiently secure in themselves that their shape and weight do not concern them so greatly. The methods used to do this vary considerably and may include various combinations of those outlined below.

Psychotherapy-based methods. The therapist develops a dynamic understanding of the patient's difficulties and may use transference as an essential element of treatment. If the psychotherapeutic approach is used on its own, the patient will not receive any direct guidance about their eating habits. Some therapists who use this approach believe that it is futile for the patient to be asked to give up their bulimic symptoms until they have understood the underlying issues causing and maintaining the behaviour.

Giving advice. This may include information about body weight regulation, the adverse effects of self-induced vomiting or laxatives, how to eat (e.g., slowly, tasting the food) and what to eat. There is considerable differences between therapist's opinions about what is appropriate dietary advice. Some recommend eating health-type foods. Others prescribe carbohydrate inclusion at each meal and aim for the patient to be able to eat binge foods normally. This issue needs to be discussed with the rest of the therapeutic team.

Behavioural methods. The behavioural methods vary and may change as treatment progresses. These include self-monitoring, giving graded goals related to what to eat and when to eat, giving rewards for not binging, and gradually increasing times when binging is avoided.

Cognitive methods. The cognitive procedures include self-monitoring, imagining the thoughts which would occur if certain difficult situations happened, techniques for improving self-esteem, training in problem-solving, measures to reduce the risk of relapse and cognitive restructuring techniques. Cognitive restructuring procedures follow four stages: (a) the identification of dysfunctional thoughts; (b) the examination of these thoughts; (c) the identification of underlying dysfunctional beliefs and values; and (d) the examination of these beliefs and values.

Usually the choice of treatment will depend on the therapist's and the team philosphy, skills and resources, and may involve working with individuals and groups and developing and coordinating self-help groups. Details of the various treatments are described by their respective proponents: e.g. Woodman (1980), Fairburn (1981, 1985), Eichenbaum and Orbach (1983), and Lacey (1983, 1985).

Occupational Therapy with Bulimia Nervosa in an Inpatient Setting

Patients in need of inpatient treatment are near the low level/personality disordered end of the spectrum of difficulties. Successful treatment depends on the patient stopping binging and vomiting and in making considerable changes in other aspects of their lives. Many will need to develop or regain confidence in their ability to engage in social activities, to eat with others, to prepare, cook and eat normal meals, to work and, perhaps crucially, to learn new ways of dealing with interpersonal relationships. They will be receiving treatment daily and there will usually be considerable opportunity for the OT to provide an extensive programme to meet these objectives. The therapist may be encouraged to develop skills in individual and group psychotherapy, cognitive methods, behavioural methods and family therapy as part of the multidisciplinary team.

Early stages. The primary aim is for the therapist to built up a good rapport with the patient to enable the difficult and often painful conflicts which have created the BN to be resolved. Initially issues of control will predominate. The patient will be struggling to accept help and participate in treatment while, at the same time, being frightened of not being in full control of the eating behaviour or emotions.

Psychodrama allows personal situations to be enacted which may clarify the ways in which control has been employed. In art therapy fears of becoming 'out of control' may be heightened by overcontrolled artwork, and/or by the patient metaphorically binging on the art materials, the space on the paper or on time. Dance or movement provide a unique opportunity for exploration of the intense desire by the patient to 'conquer the body' and additionally provide the opportunity to experience the body freely and positively.

Gradually treatment shifts towards helping the emergence of a stronger sense of 'self'. Activities which necessitate autonomy, self-direction and active participation may be useful (e.g., creative writing, poetry and art). Great fears about their own potential for destructive or violent feelings may emerge, perhaps towards the people loved or needed. Art, writing or movement can allow the expression of these feelings in a safe setting.

Middle stages. This is the time to look at the role binging has played. There may be a cycle of feelings and behaviour related to food which the bulimic person needs to break. In the cycle the person feels virtuous while they restrict their intake, but as hunger begins to dominate they feel taken over by craving for food, and guilt at these feelings. Anxiety and need build up and lead to a binge which initially gives relief, but this rapidly changes to further feelings of guilt and feelings of being ugly and repulsive which lead back to restriction. Where this cycle is entrenched, the person will have neglected their other needs, and may be unable to recognize, accept or gratify these. By making the link between the destructive food cycle and the denial of other needs explicit, the aim of breaking the cycle and learning to meet other personal needs can be added. Purging may be associated with the attempt to somehow eradicate bad feelings, whether about themselves or others. Tolerating feelings therefore becomes an essential part of their personal development.

Activities which help a person find out, express and satisfy their needs include drama groups, assertion and social skills sessions, relaxation, and social and practical activities. Alongside these activities, it is necessary to commence working on the practicalities of learning to deal with food in a new way. Planning the correct amounts to buy, coping with being in shops without buying for a binge or counting calories excessively, preparing and eating meals, eating with others and in public places are all included now. Both the practical and emotional aspects will need to be explored.

Those people with low level difficulties will need to find alternative ways to cope with their impulsive streak. Certain activities (e.g., sport or gardening) may be used to channel energy, and these can serve as precursors to insight directed activities such as art, drama movement or writing where self-understanding may be facilitated. Most OT activities involve tolerance of frustration and require some degree of impulse control. By focusing on attention to feelings within an activity, the patient may become more aware of 'what' produces the need to 'get rid' of certain feelings.

Latter Stages. At this point the therapist and patient are increasingly involved with the life which the person will be returning to. Their aims are to anticipate and resolve difficulties in domestic, social, interpersonal and work areas. Other aims are to consolidate experiences gained at earlier stages of treatment. Some people who abused alcohol may have to broaden their social network if they are not to return to their former habits. Domestic aims may include visiting home and preparing a meal, visiting friends and eating meals with them or doing the weekly shopping in the normal environment. Social aims may include changes which they want to make in friendships, family relationships and with work colleagues. These can be worked at through role plays and by using principles from social skills and assertive training. Typical examples include taking the initiative with friends and expressing feelings more directly. Equally important are aims to build up successful experiences with leisure activities. Periods of unstructured time may prove difficult to manage on leaving hospital as at these times the person may have feelings of emptiness and loneliness. There may be a temptation to avoid these uncomfortable feelings by frenetic overactivity or by a return to abusing food. Therefore, the patient needs to be able to turn to people and deal with the discomfort in other ways. These issues can be explored through the use of communication exercises, trust and assertion techniques.

The more the person is able to practise before leaving hospital and the more they can use the staff, their friends and other patients to talk about the difficulties which these exercises arouse, the more likely they will be able to cope and have a good prognosis.

Challenges to Treatment

Irregular attendance. The therapist needs to be sensitive to the factors underlying a patient's irregular attendance (even when the reasons for non-attendance are plausible) and look at the way the disruption of therapy is affecting the patient. Possible reasons include: (a) they find it difficult to say 'no' to people's demands; (b) they subordinate their own needs to the needs of others; (c) they are becoming frightened about giving up bulimia; (d) they rebel against the structure; (e) they are worried about their increasing dependence on the clinic or therapist; and (f) they make commitments which they are unable to fulfil. Depending upon the treatment method used, the therapist and patient work out appropriate graduated steps to modify behaviour, focus on the attitudes and beliefs that interfere with attendance or develop an understanding about how avoidance fits in to their way of coping in life.

Weight reducing dieting. Some patients will try to lose weight during the course of treatment. Some treatment methods insist that to conquer BN the patient needs to learn to eat ordinary meals and that the patient should not attempt to lose weight; they would make this a condition for the treatment being undertaken. Others allow the patient to eat food as they wish, concentrating on the role which food plays in the person's life and their need to modify their shape and weight and to control their food.

Help from family and friends. At times patients' progress is hindered by 'help' from their family and friends. For example, critical comments on what they eat (it's either too much or not enough), offering to cook them meals, trying to stop them binging by emotional blackmail are all rather negative. This 'help' might feature whether or not the patient has told family or friends about their bulimia.

Other methods of purging. A patient may change from one form of purging to another. For example, although they are able to stop vomiting their anxiety about their weight may lead them to substitute some other form of activity. It is this changing to other activities which may account for patients appearing to be eating normally and yet losing weight. These activities include using laxatives, slimming tablets, high fibre foods, diuretics and also excessive exercise.

Premenstrual tension and periods. Many female patients report that the urge to binge is much stronger when they are premenstrual and/or during the first few days of their period. Some patients continue to binge at this time of their cycle although stopping for the rest of the month.

Improving too soon. Some patients attend assessment interviews and from this intervention cease binging and so decide that further therapy is not necessary. Other patients stop binging after the initial interview and may also decide against further therapy. A further group stops binging almost as soon as they start treatment. It is mostly in the last group that a return to symptoms may be predicted. The patient improves because of the structure provided by the treatment. They do not invest sufficiently in the process of therapy and do not learn as effectively as others to face situations without binging. Soon after regular commitment to the clinic is over, and the imposed structures removed, the patient returns to old patterns. Sometimes, these patients will re-approach the clinic to restart treatment and often do much better the second time.

Dependence on therapist/clinic. Most patients who attend the clinic engage in some dependence on the therapist. Indeed, as was pointed out at the beginning of the chapter, without a good rapport between the therapist and the patient treatment would be less effective. Sometimes, however, the patient becomes attached to the therapist and the clinic in a less constructive way. When treatment ends, they feel empty. It is as if they have lived for the therapist and their self-value and esteem are enmeshed in the therapy. The earlier the OT can identify what is occurring, the more likely it is that this can be managed satisfactorily. The therapist should make leaving the clinic a major treatment goal.

Conclusions

This chapter has attempted to give a comprehensive introduction to AN and BN and the role of the OT. The references provide background information and details for those who wish to pursue the area further.

References

ARONSON, J.K. (1986) 'The level of object relations and severity of symptoms in the normal weight bulimic patient', *International Journal of Eating Disorders,* 5, 669–81.

BARR, E. (1980) 'The relationship between student and clinical supervisor', *British Journal of Occupational Therapy,* 9, 319–21.

BRUCH, H. (1978) *The Golden Cage: The Enigma of Anorexia Nervosa,* Cambridge, Mass., Harvard University Press.

CASEMENT, P. (1985) *On Learning from the Patient,* London, Tavistock Publications.

CRISP, A.H., NORTON, K.R.S., JURCZAK, S., BOWYER, C. and DUNCAN, S. (1985) 'A treatment approach to anorexia nervosa: 25 years on', *Journal of Psychiatric Research,* 19, 393–404.

DAVENLOO, H. (1980) *Short-term Dynamic Psychotherapy,* New York, Jason Aronson.

EICHENBAUM, L. and ORBACH, S. (1983) *Outside In: Inside Out,* Harmondsworth, Penguin.

FAIRBURN, C. (1981) 'A cognitive behavioural approach to the treatment of bulimia', *Psychological Medicine,* 11, 707–11.

FAIRBURN, C. (1985) 'Cognitive behavioural treatment for bulimia', in GARNER, D.M. and GARFINKEL, P.E. (Eds), *Handbook of Psychotherapy for Anorexia Nervosa and Bulimia,* New York, Guildford Press, pp. 160–92.

FURNHAM, A., KING, J. and PENDLETON, D. (1980) 'Establishing rapport: Interactional skills and occupational therapy', *British Journal of Occupational Therapy,* 9, 322–5.

LACEY, H.J. (1983) 'An outpatient treatment program for bulimia nervosa', *International Journal of Eating Disorders,* 2, 209–14.

LACEY, H.J. (1985) 'True-limited individual and group treatment for bulimia', in GARNER, D.M. and GARFINKEL, P.E. (Eds), *Handbook of Psychotherapy for Anorexia Nervosa and Bulimia,* New York, Guildford Press, pp. 431–51.

STERN, S. (1986) 'The dynamics of clinical management in the treatment of anorexia nervosa and bulimia: An organising theory', *International Journal of Eating Disorders,* 2, 233–54.

WOODMAN, D. (1980) *The Owl Was a Baker's Daughter,* Toronto, Inner City Books.

YOUN, M. (1984) 'Models of practice for occupational therapy', *British Journal of Occupational Therapy,* 12, 390–7.

Notes on Contributors

Jenny Bodenham, OTR, is Deputy Head Occupational Therapist at Hanham Hall Hospital, Bristol, UK.

Sheila Boyd, DipCOT, is an occupational therapist at the Royal Hospital for Sick Children, Glasgow, UK.

Mary Ann Bruce, MS, OTR/L, is Associate Professor at the University of Texas Health Science Center at San Antonio, USA. She is co-author of *Frames of Reference in Psychosocial Occupational Therapy* (1987).

Linda Burton, DipCOT, is a lecturer in the Derby School of Occupational Therapy, UK.

Laurie Campana, OTR, is an occupational therapist at the Kennedy Memorial Hospital, Massachusetts, USA.

Rachel Davis Daniels, OTR, is an occupational therapist at the Kennedy Memorial Hospital, Massachusetts, USA.

Sheena Duncan, DipCOT, works at Atkinson Morley's Hospital, London. Her specialist interests are anorexia nervosa, psychodrama and art therapy.

David Folts, OTR/L, works in a private psychiatric hospital in Virginia, USA, and has developed OT programmes for hospices in the area.

Gordon M. Giles, BA, DipCOT, OTR, has published extensively in occupational therapy and psychology journals. He now works at the Bay Area Head Recovery Center, Berkeley, California, USA and is preparing his second book.

Noomi Katz, PhD, OTR, is Assistant Professor at the School of Occupational Therapy, The Hebrew University, Jerusalem, Israel. She completed her basic occupational therapy training in Israel and her graduate studies at The University of Southern California in Los Angeles. She worked in several mental health facilities in Israel, Switzerland and Los Angeles. Her main interests and publications in occupational therapy are related to theory development, cognitive processes and evaluation in mental health and brain injured populations.

Carolyn Hatje Kaufman, OTR/L, is Rehabilitation Coordinator at the Kennedy Memorial Hospital, Massachusetts, USA.

Kathleen Griffith Hoehn, OTR, is an occupational therapist at the Sinai Day Hospital, West Bloomfield, Michigan, USA.

Diana Keable, DipCOT, BSc, now works at St Charles Hospital, London, UK. She has two articles on relaxation training published in the *British Journal of Occupational Therapy* and is currently writing a book on anxiety management techniques for therapists.

Barbara Konkol, OTR, is an occupational therapist with the DePaul Belleview Clinic, Milwaukee, USA, who specializes in working with the elderly substance abuser. She also holds a BS degree in journalism.

Terry Krupa, MEd, BSc (OT), is Assistant Coordinator of Continuing Care, Clarke Institute of Psychiatry, Toronto, Canada.

Patricia Laverdure, OTR, is an occupational therapist at the Kennedy Memorial Hospital, Massachusetts, USA

Mary Levens, DipCOT, works at Atkinson Morley's Hospital, London. Her specialist interests are eating disorders and art therapy.

Chris Lloyd, DipOT, BSc, is an occupational therapist at the Alberta Hospital, Edmonton, Canada, and has previously published in the area of forensic psychiatry.

Robin Moyer, OTR, is an occupational therapist at the Kennedy Memorial Hospital, Massachusetts, USA.

Marge Murphy, DipCOT, is a graduate in occupational therapy from the University of Toronto and has many years of experience working in mental health treatment centres in Canada, UK and the USA. During the last fifteen years she has focused on vocational rehabilitation.

Donna Schell, DipCOT, is Deputy Head Occupational Therapist at St Andrew's Hospital, UK. She has previously published on the subject of behaviour modification.

Mary Jo Schneider, MS, OTR, is Director of Restorative Services at DePaul Belleview Extended Care, Milwaukee, USA. She is also a Clinical Assistant Professor at the University of Wisconsin-Milwaukee and acts as an educator for occupational therapy students from several colleges and universities throughout the state of Wisconsin.

Derek W. Scott, BSc, was a research psychologist with the Team for the Assessment of Psychiatric Services, Friern and Claybury Hospitals, London, UK when this book was compiled. He has worked alongside occupational therapists in several UK hospitals, most notably St Andrew's Northampton. He has published in the areas of autism, alcoholism and anorexia. His book *Practical Approaches to Anorexia and Bulimia Nervosa,* is to be published in 1988. He is currently with the Department of Engineering Production, University of Birmingham, UK.

Rose Stockwell, BSc, DipCOT, is a part-time therapist at the Eating Disorders Clinic, St George's Hospital, London, and a part-time project worker for the Greenwich and Bexley Council on Alcohol, London. She is also an accredited counsellor.

Judie Taylor, DipCOT, is a lecturer in the Derby School of Occupational Therapy, UK.

John Thornton, MB, FRCP(C), is head of the Active Treatment Clinic for Schizophrenia, Clarke Institute of Psychiatry, Toronto and Assistant Professor in the Faculty of Medicine, University of Toronto.

Gill Trafford, DipCOT, is an occupational therapist at the Royal Hospital for Sick Children, Glasgow.

Judith Trevan-Hawke, DipCOT, Cert Ed, is a lecturer in the Department of Occupational Therapy, Queensland, Australia. She has published internationally in OT journals.

Index